SACRED TEXTS

# THE YOGA SUTRAS OF PATANJALI

## The Essential Yoga Texts for Spiritual Enlightenment

Translation and Introduction by
Swami Vivekananda

WATKINS PUBLISHING
LONDON

This translation of *The Yoga Sutras of Patanjali* was first published as *Raja Yoga or Conquering the Internal Nature* by Advaita Ashrama

This edition produced in 2007 for Sacred Texts,
an imprint of Watkins Publishing
Sixth Floor, Castle House, 75–76 Wells Street,
London W1T 3QH



1 3 5 7 9 10 8 6 4 2

Designed in Great Britain by Jerry Goldie
Typeset in Great Britain by Dorchester Typesetting Group
Printed and bound in Thailand by Imago

British Library Cataloguing-in-Publication data available

ISBN: 978-1-905857-03-6

www.watkinspublishing.com

# CONTENTS

# INTRODUCTION

Before going into the Yoga aphorisms I shall try to discuss one great question, upon which rests the whole theory of religion for the Yogis. It seems the consensus of opinion of the great minds of the world, and it has been nearly demonstrated by researches into physical nature, that we are the outcome and manifestation of an absolute condition, back of our present relative condition, and are going forward, to return to that absolute. This being granted, the question is: which is better, the absolute or this state? There are not wanting people who think that this manifested state is the highest state of man. Thinkers of great calibre are of the opinion that we are manifestations of undifferentiated being, and the differentiated state is higher than the absolute. They imagine that in the absolute there cannot be any quality; that it must be insensate, dull, and lifeless;

that only this life can be enjoyed and, therefore, we must cling to it. First of all we want to inquire into other solutions of life. There was an old solution that man after death remained the same; that all his good sides, minus his evil sides, remained for ever. Logically stated, that means that man's goal is the world; this world carried a stage higher, and eliminated of its evils, is the state they call heaven. This theory, on the face of it, is absurd and puerile, because it cannot be. There cannot be good without evil, nor evil without good. To live in a world where it is all good and no evil is what Sanskrit logicians call a "dream in the air". Another theory in modern times has been presented by several schools, that man's destiny is to go on always improving, always struggling towards, but never reaching the goal. This statement, though apparently very nice, is also absurd, because there is no such thing as motion in a straight line. Every motion is in a circle. If you can take up a stone, and project it into space, and then live long enough, that stone, if it meets with no obstruction, will come back exactly to your hand. A straight line, infinitely projected, must end in a circle.

Therefore, this idea that the destiny of man is progressing ever forward and forward, and never stopping, is absurd. Although extraneous to the subject, I may remark that this idea explains the ethical theory, that you must not hate, and must love. Because, just as in the case of electricity, the modern theory is that the power leaves the dynamo and completes the circle back to the dynamo, so with hate and love; they must come back to the source. Therefore do not hate anybody, because that hatred which comes out from you, must, in the long run, come back to you. If you love, that love will come back to you, completing the circle. It is as certain as can be, that every bit of hatred that goes out of the heart of a man comes back to him in full force, nothing can stop it; similarly every impulse of love comes back to him.

On other and practical grounds we see that the theory of eternal progression is untenable, for destruction is the goal of everything earthly. All our struggles and hopes and fears and joys, what will they lead to? We shall all end in death. Nothing is so certain as this. Where, then, is this motion in a straight line—this infinite progression? It is only going out to a distance, and coming back to the centre from which it started. See how, from nebulae, the sun, moon, and stars are produced; then they dissolve and go back to nebulae. The same is being done everywhere. The plant takes material from the earth, dissolves, and gives it back. Every form in this world is taken out of surrounding atoms and goes back to these atoms. It cannot be that the same law acts differently in different places. Law is uniform. Nothing is more certain than that. If this is the law of nature, it also applies to thought. Thought will dissolve and go back to its origin. Whether we will it or not, we shall have to return to our origin, which is called God, or Absolute. We all came from God, and we are all bound to go back to God. Call that by any name you like—God, Absolute, or Nature—the fact remains the same. "From whom all this universe comes out, in whom all that is born lives, and to whom all returns." This is one fact that is certain. Nature works on the same plan: what is being worked out in one sphere is repeated in millions of spheres. What you see with the planets, the same will it be with this earth, with men, and with all. The huge wave is a mighty compound of small waves, it may be of millions; the life of the whole world is a compound of millions of little lives, and the death of the whole world is the compound of the deaths of these millions of little beings.

Now the question arises: is going back to God the higher state, or not? The philosophers of the Yoga school emphatically answer that it is. They say that man's present state is a degeneration. There is no one religion on the face of the earth which says that man is an improvement. The idea is that his beginning is perfect and pure, that he degenerates until he cannot degenerate further, and that there must come a time when he shoots upward again to complete the circle. The circle must be described. However low he may go, he must ultimately take the upward bend and go back to the original source, which is God. Man comes from God in the beginning, in the middle he becomes man, and in the end he goes back to God. This is the method of putting it in the dualistic form. The monistic form is that man is God, and goes back to Him again. If our present state is the higher one, then why is there so much horror and misery, and why is there an end to it? If this is the higher state, why does it end? That which corrupts and degenerates cannot be the highest state. Why should it be so diabolical, so unsatisfying? It is only excusable, inasmuch as through it we are taking a higher groove; we have to pass through it in order to become regenerate again. Put a seed into the ground and it disintegrates, dissolves after a time, and out of that dissolution comes the splendid tree. Every soul must disintegrate to become God. So it follows that the sooner we get out of this state we call "man", the better for us. Is it by committing suicide that we get out of this state? Not at all. That will be making it worse. Torturing ourselves, or condemning the world, is not the way to get out. We have to pass through the Slough of Despond, and the sooner we are through the better. It must always be remembered that man state is not the highest state.

The really difficult part to understand is that this state, the Absolute, which has been called the highest, is not, as some fear, that of the zoophyte, or of the stone. According to them, there are only two states of existence, one of the stone, and the other of thought. What right have they to limit existence to these two? Is there not something infinitely superior to thought? The vibrations of light, when they are very low, we do not see; when they become a little more intense, they become light to us; when they become still more intense, we do not see them—it is dark to us. Is the darkness in the end the same darkness as in the beginning? Certainly not; they are different as the two poles. Is the thoughtlessness of the stone the same as the thoughtlessness of God? Certainly not. God does not think; He does not reason. Why should He? Is anything unknown to Him, that He should reason? The stone cannot reason; God does not. Such is the difference. These philosophers think it is awful if we go beyond thought; they find nothing beyond thought.

There are much higher states of existence beyond reasoning. It is really beyond the intellect that the first state of religious life is to be found. When you step beyond thought and intellect and all reasoning, then you have made the first step towards God; and that is the beginning of life. What is commonly called life is but an embryo state.

The next question will be: what proof is there that the state beyond thought and reasoning is the highest state? In the first place, all the great men of the world, much greater than those that only talk, men who moved the world, men who never thought of any selfish ends whatever, have declared that this life is but a little stage on the way towards Infinity which is beyond. In the second place, they not only say so, but show the way to everyone to explain their methods, that all can follow in their steps. In the third place, there is no other way left. There is no other explanation. Taking for granted that there is no higher state, why are we going through this circle all the time; what reason can explain the world? The sensible world will be the limit to our knowledge if we cannot go farther, if we must not ask for anything more. This is what is called agnosticism. But what reason is there to believe in the testimony of the senses? I would call that man a true agnostic who would stand still in the street and die. If reason is all in all, it leaves us no place to stand on this side of nihilism. If a man is agnostic of everything but money, fame, and name, he is only a fraud. Kant has proved beyond all doubt that we cannot penetrate beyond the tremendous dead wall called reason. But that is the very first idea upon which all Indian thought takes its stand, and dares to seek, and succeeds in finding something higher than reason, where alone the explanation of the present state is to be found. This is the value of the study of something that will take us beyond the world. "Thou art our father, and wilt take us to the other shore of this ocean of ignorance." That is the science of religion, nothing else.

## CHAPTER I

# CONCENTRATION: ITS SPIRITUAL USES

1. *Now concentration is explained.*

2. *Yoga is restraining the mind stuff (Chitta) from taking various forms (Vrittis).*

A good deal of explanation is necessary here. We have to understand what Chitta is, and what the Vrittis are. I have eyes. Eyes do not see. Take away the brain centre which is in the head, the eyes will still be there, the retinae complete, as also the pictures of objects on them, and yet the eyes will not see. So the eyes are only a secondary instrument, not the organ of vision. The organ of vision is in a nerve centre of the brain. The two eyes will not be sufficient.

Sometimes a man is asleep with his eyes open. The light is there and the picture is there, but a third thing is necessary—the mind must be joined to the organ. The eye is the external instrument; we need also the brain centre and the agency of the mind. Carriages roll down a street, and you do not hear them. Why? Because your mind has not attached itself to the organ of hearing. First, there is the instrument, then there is the organ, and third the mind attached to these two. The mind takes the impression farther in, and presents it to the determinative faculty—Buddhi—which reacts. Along with this reaction flashes the idea of egoism. Then this mixture of action and reaction is presented to the Purusha, the real Soul, who perceives an object in this mixture. The organs (Indriyas), together with the mind (Manas), the determinative faculty (Buddhi), and egoism (Ahankara), form the group called the Antakarana (the internal instrument). They are but various processes in the mind stuff, called Chitta. The waves of thought in the Chitta are called Vrittis (literally "whirlpool"). What is thought? Thought is a force, as is gravitation or repulsion. From the infinite storehouse of force in nature, the instrument called Chitta takes hold of some, absorbs it and sends it out as thought. Force is supplied to us through food, and out of that food the body obtains the power of motion, etc. Others, the finer forces, it throws out in what we call thought. So we see that the mind is not intelligent; yet it appears to be intelligent. Why? Because the intelligent soul is behind it. You are the only sentient being; mind is only the instrument through which you catch the external world. Take this book; as a book it does not exist outside; what exists outside is unknown and unknowable. The unknowable furnishes the suggestion that gives a blow to the mind, and the mind gives out the reaction in the form of a book, in the same manner as when a stone is thrown into the water, the water is thrown against it in the form of waves. The real universe is the occasion of the reaction of the mind. A book form, or an elephant form, or a man form, is not outside; all that we know is our mental reaction from the outer suggestion. "Matter is the permanent possibility of sensations," said John Stuart Mill. It is only the suggestion that is outside. Take an oyster for example. You know how pearls are made. A parasite gets inside the shell and causes irritation, and the oyster throws a sort of enamelling round it, and this makes the pearl. The universe of experience is our own enamel, so to say, and the real universe is the parasite serving as nucleus. The ordinary man will never understand it, because when he tries to do so, he throws out an enamel, and sees only his own enamel. Now we understand what is meant by these Vrittis. The real man is behind the mind; the mind is the instrument in his hands; it is his intelligence that is percolating through the mind. It is only when you stand behind the mind that it becomes intelligent. When man gives it up, it falls to pieces and is nothing. Thus you understand what is meant by Chitta. It is the mind stuff, and Vrittis are the waves and ripples rising in it when external causes impinge on it. These Vrittis are our universe.

The bottom of a lake we cannot see, because its surface is covered with ripples. It is only possible for us to catch a glimpse of the bottom, when the ripples have subsided, and the water is calm. If the water is muddy or is agitated all the time, the bottom will not be seen. If it is clear, and there are no waves, we shall see the bottom. The bottom of the lake is our own true Self; the lake is the Chitta and the waves the Vrittis. Again, the mind is in three states, one of which is darkness, called Tamas, found in brutes and idiots; it only acts to injure. No other idca comes into that state of mind. Then there is the active state of mind, Rajas, whose chief motives are power and enjoyment. "I will be powerful and rule others." Then there is the state called Sattva, serenity, calmness, in which the waves cease, and the water of the mind lake becomes clear. It is not inactive, but rather intensely active. It is the greatest manifestation of power to be calm. It is easy to be active. Let the reins go, and the horses will run away with you. Anyone can do that, but he who can stop the plunging horses is the strong man. Which requires the greater strength, letting go or restraining? The calm man is not the man who is dull. You must not mistake Sattva for dullness or laziness. The calm man is the one who has control over the mind waves. Activity is the manifestation of inferior strength, and calmness of the superior.

The Chitta is always trying to get back to its natural pure state, but the organs draw it out. To restrain it, to check this outward tendency, and to start it on the return journey to the essence of intelligence is the first step in Yoga, because only in this way can the Chitta get into its proper course.

Although the Chitta is in every animal, from the lowest to the highest, it is only in the human form that we find it as the intellect. Until the mind stuff can take the form of intellect it is not possible for it to return through all these steps, and liberate the soul. Immediate salvation is impossible for the cow or the dog, although they have mind, because their Chitta cannot as yet take that form which we call intellect.

The Chitta manifests itself in the following forms—scattering, darkening, gathering, one-pointed, and concentrated. The scattering form is activity. Its tendency is to manifest in the form of pleasure or of pain. The darkening form is dullness which tends to injury. The commentator says, the third form is natural to the Devas, the angels, and the first and second to the demons. The gathering form is when it struggles to centre itself. The one-pointed form is when it tries to concentrate, and the concentrated form is what brings us to Samadhi.

3. *At that time (the time of concentration) the seer (Purusha) rests in his own (unmodified) state.*

As soon as the waves have stopped, and the lake has become quiet, we see its bottom. So with the mind; when it is calm, we see what our own nature is; we do not mix ourselves but remain our own selves.

4. *At other times (other than that of concentration) the seer is identified with the modifications.*

For instance, someone blames me; this produces a modification, Vritti, in my mind, and I identify myself with it, and the result is misery.

5. *There are five classes of modifications, (some) painful and (others) not painful.*

6. *(These are) right knowledge, indiscrimination, verbal delusion, sleep and memory.*

7. *Direct perception, inference and competent evidence are proofs.*

When two of our perceptions do not contradict each other, we call it proof. I hear something, and if it contradicts something already perceived, I begin to fight it out, and do not believe it. There are also three kinds of proof. Direct perception, Pratyaksha, whatever we see and feel, is proof, if there has been nothing to delude the senses. I see the world; that is sufficient proof that it exists. Secondly, Anumana, inference; you see a sign, and from the sign you come to the thing signified. Thirdly, Aptavakya, the direct evidence of the Yogis, of those who have seen the truth. We are all of us struggling towards knowledge. But you and I have to struggle hard, and come to knowledge through a long tedious process of reasoning, but the Yogi, the pure one, has gone beyond all this. Before his mind, the past, the present, and the future are alike, one book for him to read; he does not require to go through the tedious processes for knowledge we have to; his words are proof, because he sees knowledge in himself. These, for instance, are the authors of the sacred scriptures; therefore the scriptures are proof. If any such persons are living now their words will be proof. Other philosophers go into long discussions about Aptavakya and they say, "What is the proof of their words?" The proof is their direct perception. Because whatever I see is proof, and whatever you see is proof, if it does not contradict any past knowledge. There is knowledge beyond the senses, and whenever it does not contradict reason and past human experience, that knowledge is proof. Any madman may come into this room and say he sees angels around him; that would not be proof. In the first place, it must be true knowledge; and secondly, it must not contradict past knowledge; and thirdly, it must depend upon the character of the man who gives it out. I hear it said that the character of the man is not of so much importance as what he may say: we must first hear what he says. This may be true in other things. A man may be wicked, and yet make an astronomical discovery, but in religion it is different, because no impure man will ever have the power to reach the truths of religion. Therefore we have first of all to see that the man who declares himself to be an Apta is a perfectly unselfish and holy person; secondly, that he has reached beyond the senses; and thirdly, that what he says does not contradict the past knowledge of humanity. Any new discovery of truth does not contradict the past truth, but fits into it. And fourthly, that truth must have a possibility of verification. If a man says, "I have seen a vision", and tells me that I have no right to see it, I believe him not. Everyone must have the power to see it for himself. No one who sells his knowledge is an Apta. All these conditions must be fulfilled; you must first see that the man is pure, and that he has no selfish motive: that he has no thirst for gain or fame. Secondly, he must show that he is superconscious. He must give us something that we cannot get from our senses, and which is for the benefit of the world. Thirdly, we must see that it does not contradict other truths; if it contradicts other scientific truths, reject it at once. Fourthly, the man should never be singular; he should only represent what all men can attain. The three sorts of proof are, then, direct sense perception, inference, and the words of an Apta. I cannot translate this word into English. It is not the word "inspired", because inspiration is believed to come from outside, while this knowledge comes from the man himself. The literal meaning is "attained".

8. *Indiscrimination is false knowledge not established in real nature.*

The next class of Vrittis that arises is mistaking one thing for another, as a piece of mother-of-pearl is taken for a piece of silver.

9. *Verbal delusion follows from words having no (corresponding) reality.*

There is another class of Vrittis called Vikalpa. A word is uttered, and we do not wait to consider its meaning; we jump to a conclusion immediately. It is the sign of weakness of the Chitta. Now you can understand the theory of restraint. The weaker the man, the less he has of restraint. Examine yourselves always by that test. When you are going to be angry or miserable, reason it out how it is that some news that has come to you is throwing your mind into Vrittis.

10. *Sleep is a Vritti which embraces the feeling of voidness.*

The next class of Vrittis is called sleep and dream. When we awake, we know that we have been sleeping; we can only have memory of perception. That which we do not perceive we never can have any memory of. Every reaction is a wave in the lake. Now, if, during sleep, the mind had no waves, it would have no perceptions, positive or negative, and, therefore, we would not remember them. The very reason of our remembering sleep is that during sleep there was a certain class of waves in the mind. Memory is another class of Vrittis which is called Smriti.

11. *Memory is when the (Vrittis of) perceived subjects do not slip away (and through impressions come back to consciousness).*

Memory can come from direct perception, false knowledge, verbal delusion, and sleep. For instance, you hear a word. That word is like a stone thrown into the lake of the Chitta; it causes a ripple, and that ripple rouses a series of ripples; this is memory. So in sleep. When the peculiar kind of ripple called sleep throws the Chitta into a ripple of memory, it is called a dream. Dream is another form of the ripple which in the waking state is called memory.

12. *Their control is by practice and non-attachment.*

The mind, to have non-attachment, must be clear, good and rational. Why should we practise? Because each action is like the pulsations quivering over the surface of the lake. The vibration dies out, and what is left? The Sanskaras, the impressions. When a large number of these impressions is left on the mind, they coalesce and become a habit. It is said, "Habit is second nature"; it is first nature also, and the whole nature of man; everything that we are is the result of habit. That gives us consolation, because, if it is only habit, we can make and unmake it at any time. The Sanskaras are left by these vibrations passing out of our mind, each one of them leaving its result. Our character is the sum total of these marks, and according as some particular wave prevails, one takes that tone. If good prevails, one becomes good; if wickedness, one becomes wicked; if joyfulness, one becomes happy. The only remedy for bad habits is counter habits; all the bad habits that have left their impressions are to be controlled by good habits. Go on doing good, thinking holy thoughts continuously; that is the only way to suppress base impressions. Never say any man is hopeless, because he only represents a character, a bundle of habits, which can be checked by new and better ones. Character is repeated habits, and repeated habits alone can reform character.

13. *Continuous struggle to keep them (the Vrittis) perfectly restrained is practice.*

What is practice? The attempt to restrain the mind in Chitta form, to prevent its going out into waves.

14. *It becomes firmly grounded by long constant efforts with great love (for the end to be attained).*

Restraint does not come in one day, but by long continued practice.

15. *That effect which comes to those who have given up their thirst after objects, either seen or heard, and which wills to control the objects, is non-attachment.*

The two motive powers of our actions are (1) what we see ourselves, (2) the experience of others. These two forces throw the mind, the lake, into various waves. Renunciation is the power of battling against these forces and holding the mind in check. Their renunciation is what we want. I am passing through a street, and a man comes and takes away my watch. That is my own experience. I see it myself, and it immediately throws my Chitta into a wave, taking the form of anger. Allow not that to come. If you cannot prevent that, you are nothing; if you can, you have Vairagya. Again, the experience of the worldly minded teaches us that sense enjoyments are the highest ideal. These are tremendous temptations. To deny them, and not allow the mind to come to a wave form with regard to them, is renunciation; to control the twofold motive powers arising from my own experience and from the experience of others, and thus prevent the Chitta from being governed by them, is Vairagya. These should be controlled by me, and not I by them. This sort of mental strength is called renunciation. Vairagya is the only way to freedom.

16. *That is extreme non-attachment which gives up even the qualities, and comes from the knowledge of (the real nature of) the Purusha.*

It is the highest manifestation of the power of Vairagya when it takes away even our attraction towards the qualities. We have first to understand what the Purusha, the Self is, and what the qualities are. According to Yoga philosophy, the whole of nature consists of three qualities or forces; one is called Tamas, another Rajas, and the third Sattva. These three qualities manifest themselves in the physical world as darkness or inactivity, attraction or repulsion and equilibrium of the two. Everything that is in nature, all manifestations, are combinations and recombinations of these three forces. Nature has been divided into various categories by the Sankhyas; the Self of man is beyond all these, beyond nature. It is effulgent, pure and perfect. Whatever of intelligence we see in nature is but the reflection of this Self upon nature. Nature itself is insentient. You must remember that the word nature also includes the mind; mind is in nature; thought is in nature; from thought, down to the grossest form of matter, everything is in nature, the manifestation of nature. This nature has covered the Self of man, and when nature takes away the covering, the Self appears in Its own glory. The non-attachment, as described in aphorism 15 (as being control of objects or nature) is the greatest help towards manifesting the Self. The next aphorism defines Samadhi, perfect concentration, which is the goal of the Yogi.

17. *The concentration called right knowledge is that which is followed by reasoning, discrimination, bliss, unqualified egoism.*

Samadhi is divided into two varieties. One is called the Samprajnata, and the other the Asamprajnata. In the Samprajnata Samadhi come all the powers of controlling nature. It is of four varieties. The first variety is called the Savitarka, when the mind meditates upon an object again and again by isolating it from other objects. There are two sorts of objects for meditation in the twenty-five categories of the Sankhyas: (1) the twenty-four insentient categories of nature, and (2) the one sentient Purusha. This part of Yoga is based entirely on Sankhya philosophy, about which I have already told you. As you will remember, egoism and will and mind have a common basis—the Chitta or the mind stuff—out of which they are all manufactured. The mind stuff takes in the forces of nature, and projects them as thought. There must be something, again, where both force and matter are one. This is called Avyakta, the unmanifested state of nature before creation, and to which, after the end of a cycle, the whole of nature returns, to come out again after another period. Beyond that is the Purusha, the essence of intelligence. Knowledge is power, and as soon as we begin to know a thing, we get power over it; so also when the mind begins to meditate on the different elements, it gains power over them. That sort of meditation where the external gross elements are the objects is called Savitarka. Vitarka means question; Savitarka, with question, questioning the elements, as it were, that they may give their truths and their powers to the man who meditates upon them. There is no liberation in getting powers. It is a worldly search after enjoyments, and there is no enjoyment in this life; all search for enjoyment is vain; that is the old, old lesson which man finds so hard to learn. When he does learn it, he gets out of the universe and becomes free. The possession of what are called occult powers is only intensifying the world, and in the end, intensifying suffering. Though as a scientist, Patanjali is bound to point out the possibilities of this science, he never misses an opportunity to warn us against these powers.

Again, in the very same meditation, when one struggles to take the elements out of time and space, and think of them as they are, it is called Nirvitarka, without question. When the meditation goes a step higher, and takes the Tanmatras as its object, and thinks of them as in time and space, it is called Savichara, with discrimination; and when in the same meditation one eliminates time and space, and thinks of the fine elements as they are, it is called Nirvichara, without discrimination. The next step is when the elements are given up, both gross and fine, and the object of meditation is the interior organ, the thinking organ. When the thinking organ is thought of as bereft of the qualities of activity and dullness, it is then called Sananda, the blissful Samadhi. When the mind itself is the object of meditation, when meditation becomes very ripe and concentrated, when all ideas of the gross and fine materials are given up, when the Sattva state only of the ego remains, but differentiated from all other objects, it is called Sasmita Samadhi. The man who has attained to this has attained to what is called in the Vedas "bereft of body". He can think of himself as without his gross body; but he will have to think of himself as with a fine body. Those that in this state get merged in nature without attaining the goal are called Prakritilayas, but those who do not stop even there reach the goal, which is freedom.

18. *There is another Samadhi which is attained by the constant practice of cessation of all mental activity, in which the Chitta retains only the unmanifested impressions.*

This is the perfect superconscious Asamprajnata Samadhi, the state which gives us freedom. The first state does not give us freedom, does not liberate the soul. A man may attain to all powers, and yet fall again. There is no safeguard until the soul goes beyond nature. It is very difficult to do so, although the method seems easy. The method is to meditate on the mind itself, and whenever thought comes, to strike it down, allowing no thought to come into the mind, thus making it an entire vacuum. When we can really do this, that very moment we shall attain liberation. When persons without training and preparation try to make their minds vacant, they are likely to succeed only in covering themselves with Tamas, the material of ignorance, which makes the mind dull and stupid, and leads them to think that they are making a vacuum of the mind. To be able to really do that is to manifest the greatest strength, the highest control. When this state, Asamprajnata, superconsciousness, is reached, the Samadhi becomes seedless. What is meant by that? In a concentration where there is consciousness, where the mind succeeds only in quelling the waves in the Chitta and holding them down, the waves remain in the form of tendencies. These tendencies (of seeds) become waves again, when the time comes. But when you have destroyed all these tendencies, almost destroyed the mind, then the Samadhi becomes seedless, there are no more seeds in the mind out of which to manufacture again and again this plant of life, this ceaseless round of birth and death.

You may ask, what state would that be in which there is no mind, there is no knowledge? What we call knowledge is a lower state than the one beyond knowledge. You must always bear in mind that the extremes look very much alike. If a very low vibration of ether is taken as darkness, an intermediate state as light, very high vibration will be darkness again. Similarly, ignorance is the lowest state, knowledge is the middle state, and beyond knowledge is the highest state, the two extremes of which seem the same. Knowledge itself is a manufactured something, a combination; it is not reality.

What is the result of constant practice of this higher concentration? All old tendencies of restlessness and dullness will be destroyed, as well as the tendencies of goodness too. The case is similar to that of the chemicals used to take the dirt and alloy off gold. When the ore is smelted down, the dross is burnt along with the chemicals. So this constant controlling power will stop the previous bad tendencies, and eventually, the good ones also. Those good and evil tendencies will suppress each other, leaving alone the Soul in its own splendour, untrammelled by either good or bad, the omnipresent, omnipotent, and omniscient. Then the man will know that he had neither birth nor death, nor need of heaven or earth. He will know that he neither came nor went, it was nature which was moving, and that movement was reflected upon the Soul. The form of the light reflected by the glass upon the wall moves, and the wall foolishly thinks it is moving. So with all of us; it is the Chitta constantly moving making itself into various forms, and we think that we are these various forms. All these delusions will vanish. When that free Soul will command—not pray or beg, but command—then whatever it desires will be immediately fulfilled; whatever it wants it will be able to do. According to the Sankhya philosophy, there is no God. It says that there can be no God of this universe, because if there were one, He must be a soul, and a soul must be either bound or free. How can the soul that is bound by nature, or controlled by nature, create? It is itself a slave. On the other hand, why should the Soul that is free create and manipulate all these things? It has no desires, so it cannot have any need to create. Secondly, it says the theory of God is an unnecessary one; nature explains all. What is the use of any God? But Kapila teaches that there are many souls, who, though nearly attaining perfection, fall short because they cannot perfectly renounce all powers. Their minds for a time merge in nature, to re-emerge as its masters. Such gods there are. We shall all become such gods, and according to the Sankhyas, the God spoken of in the Vedas really means one of these free souls. Beyond them there is not an eternally free and blessed Creator of the universe. On the other hand, the Yogis say, "Not so, there is a God, there is one Soul separate from all other souls, and He is the eternal Master of all creation, the ever free, the Teacher of all teachers." The Yogis admit that those, whom the Sankhyas call "the merged in nature", also exist. They are Yogis who have fallen short of perfection, and though, for a time debarred from attaining the goal, remain as rulers of parts of the universe.

19. *(This Samadhi when not followed by extreme non-attachment) becomes the cause of the remanifestation of the gods and of those that become merged in nature.*

20. *To others (this Samadhi) comes through faith, energy, memory, concentration, and discrimination of the real.*

These are they who do not want the position of gods or even that of rulers of cycles. They attain to liberation.

21. *Success is speedy for the extremely energetic.*

22. *The success of Yogis differs according as the means they adopt are mild, medium, or intense.*

23. *Or by devotion to Ishvara.*

24. *Ishvara (the Supreme Ruler) is a special Purusha, untouched by misery, actions, their results, and desires.*

We must again remember that the Patanjali Yoga philosophy is based upon the Sankhya philosophy; only in the latter there is no place for God, while with the Yogis God has a place. The Yogis, however, do not mention many ideas about God, such as creating. God as the Creator of thc universe is not meant by the Ishvara of the Yogis. According to the Vedas, Ishvara is the Creator of the universe; because it is harmonious, it must be the manifestation of one will. The Yogis want to establish a God, but they arrive at Him in a peculiar fashion of their own. They say:

25. *In Him becomes infinite that all-knowingness which in others is (only) a germ.*

The mind must always travel between two extremes. You can think of limited space, but that very idea gives you also unlimited space. Close your eyes and think of a little space; at the same time that you perceive the little circle, you have a circle round it of unlimited dimensions. It is the same with time. Try to think of a second; you will have, with the same act of perception, to think of time which is unlimited. So with knowledge. Knowledge is only a germ in man, but you will have to think of infinite knowledge around it, so that the very constitution of our mind shows us that there is unlimited knowledge, and the Yogis call that unlimited knowledge God.

26. *He is the Teacher of even the ancient teachers, being not limited by time.*

It is true that all knowledge is within ourselves, but this has to be called forth by another knowledge. Although the capacity to know is inside us, it must be called out, and that calling out of knowledge can only be done, a Yogi maintains, through another knowledge. Dead, insentient matter never calls out knowledge, it is the action of knowledge that brings out knowledge. Knowing beings must be with us to call forth what is in us, so these teachers were always necessary. The world was never without them, and no knowledge can come without them. God is the Teacher of all teachers, because these teachers, however great they may have been—gods or angels—were all bound and limited by time, while God is not. There are two peculiar deductions of the Yogis. The first is that in thinking of the limited, the mind must think of the unlimited; and that if one part of that perception is true, so also must the other be, for the reason that their value as perceptions of the mind is equal. The very fact that man has a little knowledge shows that God has unlimited knowledge. If I am to take one, why not the other? Reason forces me to take both or reject both. If I believe that there is a man with a little knowledge, I must also admit that there is someone behind him with unlimited knowledge. The second deduction is that no knowledge can come without a teacher. It is true as the modern philosophers say, that there is something in man which evolves out of him; all knowledge is in man, but certain environments are necessary to call it out. We cannot find any knowledge without teachers. If there are men teachers, god teachers, or angel teachers, they are all limited; who was the teacher before them? We are forced to admit, as a last conclusion, one teacher, who is not limited by time; and that One Teacher of infinite knowledge, without beginning or end, is called God.

27. *His manifesting word is Om.*

Every idea that you have in the mind has a counterpart in a word; the word and the thought are inseparable. The external part of one and the same thing is what we call word, and the internal part is what we call thought. No man can, by analysis, separate thought from word. The idea that language was created by men—certain men sitting together and deciding upon words, has been proved to be wrong. So long as man has existed there have been words and language. What is the connection between an idea and a word? Although we see that there must always be a word with a thought, it is not necessary that the same thought requires the same word. The thought may be the same in twenty different countries, yet the language is different. We must have a word to express each thought, but these words need not necessarily have the same sound. Sounds will vary in different nations. Our commentator says, "Although the relation between thought and word is perfectly natural, yet it does not mean a rigid connection between one sound and one idea." These sounds vary, yet the relation between the sounds and the thoughts is a natural one. The connection between thoughts and sounds is good only if there be a real connection between the thing signified and the symbol; until then that symbol will never come into general use. A symbol is the manifester of the thing signified, and if the thing signified has already an existence, and if, by experience, we know that the symbol has expressed that thing many times, then we are sure that there is a real relation between them. Even if the things are not present, there will be thousands who will know them by their symbols. There must be a natural connection between the symbol and the thing signified; then, when that symbol is pronounced, it recalls the thing signified. The commentator says the manifesting word of God is Om. Why does he emphasize this word? There are hundreds of words for God. One thought is connected with a thousand words; the idea "God" is connected with hundreds of words, and each one stands as a symbol for God. Very good. But there must be a generalization among all these words, some substratum, some common ground of all these symbols, and that which is the common symbol will be the best, and will really represent them all. In making a sound we use the larynx and the palate as a sounding board. Is there any material sound of which all other sounds must be manifestations, one which is the most natural sound? Om (AUM) is such a sound, the basis of all sound. The first letter, *A*, is the root sound, the key, pronounced without touching any part of the tongue or palate; *M* represents the last sound in the series, being produced by the closed lips, and the *U* rolls from the very root to the end of the sounding board of the mouth. Thus, Om represents the whole phenomena of sound producing. As such, it must be the natural symbol, the matrix of all the various sounds. It denotes the whole range and possibility of all the words that can be made. Apart from these speculations, we see that around this word Om are centred all the different religious ideas in India; all the various religious ideas of the Vedas have gathered themselves round this word Om. What has that to do with America and England, or any other country? Simply this, that the word has been retained at every stage of religious growth in India, and it has been manipulated to mean all the various ideas about God.

Monists, dualists, monodualists, separatists, and even atheists took up this Om. Om has become the one symbol for the religious aspiration of the vast majority of human beings. Take, for instance, the English word God. It covers only a limited function, and if you go beyond it, you have to add adjectives, to make it personal, or impersonal, or Absolute God. So with the words for God in every other language; their signification is very small. This word Om, however, has around it all the various significances. As such it should be accepted by everyone.

28. *The repetition of this (Om) and meditating on its meaning (is the way).*

Why should there be repetition? We have not forgotten the theory of Sanskaras, that the sum total of impressions lives in the mind. They become more and more latent but remain there, and as soon as they get the right stimulus, they come out. Molecular vibration never ceases. When this universe is destroyed, all the massive vibrations disappear; the sun, moon, stars, and earth, melt down; but the vibrations remain in the atoms. Each atom performs the same function as the big worlds do. So even when the vibrations of the Chitta subside, its molecular vibrations go on, and when they get the impulse, come out again. We can now understand what is meant by repetition. It is the greatest stimulus that can be given to the spiritual Sanskaras. "One moment of company with the holy makes a ship to cross this ocean of life." Such is the power of association. So this repetition of Om, and thinking of its meaning, is keeping good company in your own mind. Study, and then meditate on what you have studied. Thus light will come to you, the Self will become manifest.

But one must think of Om, and of its meaning too. Avoid evil company, because the scars of old wounds are in you, and evil company is just the thing that is necessary to call them out. In the same way we are told that good company will call out the good impressions that are in us, but which have become latent. There is nothing holier in the world than to keep good company, because the good impressions will then tend to come to the surface.

29. *From that is gained (the knowledge of) introspection, and the destruction of obstacles.*

The first manifestation of the repetition and thinking of Om is that the introspective power will manifest more and more, all the mental and physical obstacles will begin to vanish. What are the obstacles to the Yogi?

30. *Disease, mental laziness, doubt, lack of enthusiasm, lethargy, clinging to sense enjoyments, false perception, non-attaining concentration, and falling away from the state when obtained, are the obstructing distractions.*

*Disease*. This body is the boat which will carry us to the other shore of the ocean of life. It must be taken care of. Unhealthy persons cannot be Yogis. *Mental laziness* makes us lose all lively interest in the subject, without which there will neither be the will nor the energy to practise. *Doubts* will arise in the mind about the truth of the science, however strong one's intellectual conviction may be, until certain peculiar psychic experiences come, as hearing or seeing at a distance, etc. These glimpses strengthen the mind and make the student persevere. *Falling away . . . when obtained.* Some days or weeks when you are practising, the mind will be calm and easily concentrated, and you will find yourself progressing fast. All of a sudden the progress will stop one day, and you will find yourself, as it were, stranded. Persevere. All progress proceeds by such rise and fall.

31. *Grief, mental distress, tremor of the body, irregular breathing accompany non-retention of concentration.*

Concentration will bring perfect repose to mind and body every time it is practised. When the practice has been misdirected, or not enough controlled, these disturbances come. Repetition of Om and self-surrender to the Lord will strengthen the mind, and bring fresh energy. The nervous shakings will come to almost everyone. Do not mind them at all, but keep on practising. Practice will cure them, and make the seat firm.

32. *To remedy this, the practice of one subject (should be made).*

Making the mind take the form of one object for some time will destroy these obstacles. This is general advice. In the following aphorisms it will be expanded and particularized. As one practice cannot suit everyone, various methods will be advanced, and everyone by actual experience will find out that which helps him most.

33. *Friendship, mercy, gladness, and indifference, being thought of in regard to subjects, happy, unhappy, good, and evil respectively, pacify the Chitta.*

We must have these four sorts of ideas. We must have friendship for all; we must be merciful towards those that are in misery; when people are happy, we ought to be happy; and to the wicked we must be indifferent. So with all subjects that come before us. If the subject is a good one, we shall feel friendly towards it; if the subject of thought is one that is miserable, we must be merciful towards it. If it is good, we must be glad; if it is evil, we must be indifferent. These attitudes of the mind towards the different subjects that come before it will make the mind peaceful. Most of our difficulties in our daily lives come from being unable to hold our minds in this way. For instance, if a man does evil to us, instantly we want to react with evil, and every reaction of evil shows that we are not able to hold the Chitta down; it comes out in waves towards the object, and we lose our power. Every reaction in the form of hatred or evil is so much loss to the mind; and every evil thought or deed of hatred, or any thought of reaction, if it is controlled, will be laid in our favour. It is not that we lose by thus restraining ourselves; we are gaining infinitely more than we suspect. Each time we suppress hatred, or a feeling of anger, it is so much good energy stored up in our favour; that piece of energy will be converted into the higher powers.

34. *By throwing out and restraining the breath.*

The word used is Prana. Prana is not exactly breath. It is the name for the energy that is in the universe.

Whatever you see in the universe, whatever moves or works, or has life, is a manifestation of this Prana. The sum total of the energy displayed in the universe is called Prana. This Prana, before a cycle begins, remains in an almost motionless state; and when the cycle begins, this Prana begins to manifest itself. It is this Prana that is manifested as motion—as the nervous motion in human beings or animals; and the same Prana is manifesting as thought, and so on. The whole universe is a combination of Prana and Akasha; so is the human body. Out of Akasha you get the different materials that you feel and see, and out of Prana all the various forces. Now this throwing out and restraining the Prana is what is called Pranayama. Patanjali, the father of the Yoga philosophy, does not give very many particular directions about Pranayama, but later on other Yogis found out various things about this Pranayama, and made of it a great science. With Patanjali it is one of the many ways, but he does not lay much stress on it. He means that you simply throw the air out, and draw it in, and hold it for some time, that is all, and by that, the mind will become a little calmer. But, later on, you will find that out of this is evolved a particular science called Pranayama. We shall hear a little of what these later Yogis have to say.

Some of this I have told you before, but a little repetition will serve to fix it in your minds. First, you must remember that this Prana is not the breath; but that which causes the motion of the breath, that which is the vitality of the breath is the Prana. Again, the word Prana is used for all the senses; they are all called Pranas, the mind is called Prana; and so we see that Prana is force. And yet we cannot call it force, because force is only the manifestation of it. It is that which manifests itself as force and everything else in the way of motion. The Chitta, the mind stuff, is the engine which draws in the Prana from the surroundings, and manufactures out of Prana the various vital forces—those that keep the body in preservation—and thought, will, and all other powers. By the above-mentioned process of breathing we can control all the various motions in the body, and the various nerve currents that are running through the body. First we begin to recognize them, and then we slowly get control over them.

Now, these later Yogis consider that there are three main currents of this Prana in the human body. One they call Ida, another Pingala, and the third Sushumna. Pingala, according to them, is on the right side of the spinal column, and the Ida on the left, and in the middle of the spinal column is the Sushumna, an empty channel. Ida and Pingala, according to them, are the currents working in every man, and through these currents, we are performing all the functions of life. Sushumna is present in all, as a possibility; but it works only in the Yogi. You must remember that Yoga changes the body. As you go on practising, your body changes; it is not the same body that you had before the practice. That is very rational, and can be explained, because every new thought that we have must make, as it were, a new channel through the brain, and that explains the tremendous conservatism of human nature. Human nature likes to run through the ruts that are already there, because it is easy. If we think, just for example's sake, that the mind is like a needle, and the brain substance a soft lump before it, then each thought that we have makes a street, as it were, in the brain, and this street would close up, but for the grey matter which comes and makes a lining to keep it separate. If there were no grey matter, there would be no memory, because memory means going over these old streets, retracing a thought as it were. Now perhaps you have marked that when one talks on subjects in which one takes a few ideas that are familiar to everyone, and combines and recombines them, it is easy to follow because these channels are present in everyone's brain, and it is only necessary to refer to them. But whenever a new subject comes, new channels have to be made, so it is not understood readily. And that is why the brain (it is the brain, and not the people themselves) refuses unconsciously to be acted upon by new ideas. It resists. The Prana is trying to make new channels, and the brain will not allow it. This is the secret of conservatism. The fewer channels there have been in the brain, and the less the needle of the Prana has made these passages, the more conservative will be the brain, the more it will struggle against new thoughts. The more thoughtful the man, the more complicated will be the streets in his brain, and the more easily he will take to new ideas, and understand them. So with every fresh idea, we make a new impression in the brain, cut new channels through the brain stuff, and that is why we find that in the practice of Yoga (it being an entirely new set of thoughts and motives) there is so much physical resistance at first. That is why we find that the part of religion which deals with the world side of nature is so widely accepted, while the other part, the philosophy, or the psychology, which deals with the inner nature of man, is so frequently neglected.

We must remember the definition of this world of ours; it is only the Infinite Existence projected into the plane of consciousness. A little of the Infinite is projected into consciousness, and that we call our world. So there is an Infinite beyond; and religion has to deal with both—with the little lump we call our world, and with the Infinite beyond. Any religion which deals with one only of these two will be defective. It must deal with both. The part of religion which deals with the part of the Infinite which has come into the plane of consciousness, got itself caught, as it were, in the plane of consciousness, in the cage of time, space, and causation, is quite familiar to us, because we are in that already, and ideas about this world have been with us almost from time immemorial. The part of religion which deals with the Infinite beyond comes entirely new to us, and getting ideas about it produces new channels in the brain, disturbing the whole system, and that is why you find in the practice of Yoga ordinary people are at first turned out of their grooves. In order to lessen these disturbances as much as possible, all these methods are devised by Patanjali, that we may practise any one of them best suited to us.

35. *Those forms of concentration that bring extraordinary sense perceptions cause perseverance of the mind.*

This naturally comes with Dharana, concentration; the Yogis say, if the mind becomes concentrated on the tip of the nose, one begins to smell, after a few days, wonderful perfumes. If it becomes concentrated at the root of the tongue, one begins to hear sounds; if on the tip of the tongue, one begins to taste wonderful flavours; if on the middle of the tongue, one feels as if one were coming in contact with something. If one concentrates one's mind on the palate, one begins to see peculiar things. If a man whose mind is disturbed wants to take up some of these practices of Yoga, yet doubts the truth of them, he will have his doubts set at rest when, after a little practice, these things come to him, and he will persevere.

36. *Or (by the meditation on) the Effulgent Light, which is beyond all sorrow.*

This is another sort of concentration. Think of the lotus of the heart, with petals downwards, and running through it, the Sushumna; take in the breath, and while throwing the breath out imagine that the lotus is turned with the petals upwards, and inside that lotus is an effulgent light. Meditate on that.

37. *Or (by meditation on) the heart that has given up all attachment to sense objects.*

Take some holy person, some great person whom you revere, some saint whom you know to be perfectly non-attached, and think of his heart. That heart has become non-attached, and meditate on that heart; it will calm the mind. If you cannot do that, there is the next way.

38. *Or by meditating on the knowledge that comes in sleep.*

Sometimes a man dreams that he has seen angels coming to him and talking to him, that he is in an ecstatic condition, that he has heard music floating through the air. He is in a blissful condition in that dream, and when he wakes, it makes a deep impression on him. Think of that dream as real, and meditate upon it. If you cannot do that, meditate on any holy thing that pleases you.

39. *Or by the meditation on anything that appeals to one as good.*

This does not mean any wicked subject, but anything good that you like, any place that you like best, any scenery that you like best, any idea that you like best, anything that will concentrate the mind.

40. *The Yogi's mind thus meditating, becomes unobstructed from the atomic to the infinite.*

The mind, by this practice, easily contemplates the most minute, as well as the biggest thing. Thus the mind waves become fainter.

41. *The Yogi whose Vrittis have thus become powerless (controlled) obtains in the receiver, (the instrument of) receiving, and the received (the Self, the mind, and external objects), concentratedness and sameness, like the crystal (before different coloured objects).*

What results from this constant meditation? We must remember how in a previous aphorism Patanjali went into the various states of meditation, how the first would be the gross, the second the fine, and from them the advance was to still finer objects. The result of these meditations is that we can meditate as easily on the fine as on the gross objects. Here the Yogi sees the three things—the receiver, the received, and the receiving instrument—corresponding to the Soul, external objects, and the mind. There are three objects of meditation given us. First, the gross things, as bodies, or material objects; second, fine things, as the mind, the Chitta; and third, the Purusha qualified, not the Purusha itself, but the egoism. By practice, the Yogi gets established in all these meditations. Whenever he meditates he can keep out all other thoughts he becomes identified with that on which he meditates. When he meditates, he is like a piece of crystal. Before flowers the crystal becomes almost identified with the flowers. If the flower is red, the crystal looks red, or if the flower is blue, the crystal looks blue.

42. *Sound, meaning, and resulting knowledge, being mixed up, is (called) Samadhi with question.*

Sound here means vibration, meaning the nerve currents which conduct it; and knowledge, reaction. All the various meditations we have had so far, Patanjali calls Savitarka (meditation with question). Later on he gives us higher and higher Dhyanas. In these that are called "with question," we keep the duality of subject and object, which results from the mixture of word, meaning, and knowledge. There is first the external vibration, the word. This carried inward by the sense currents, is the meaning. After that there comes a reactionary wave in the Chitta, which is knowledge, but the mixture of these three makes up what we call knowledge. In all the meditations up to this we get this mixture as objects of meditation. The next Samadhi is higher.

43. *The Samadhi called "without question" (comes) when the memory is purified, or devoid of qualities, expressing only the meaning (of the meditated object).*

It is by the practice of meditation of these three that we come to the state where these three do not mix. We can get rid of them. We will first try to understand what these three are. Here is the Chitta; you will always remember the simile of the mind stuff to a lake and the vibration, the word, the sound, like a pulsation coming over it. You have that calm lake in you, and I pronounce a word, "cow". As soon as it enters through your ears there is a wave produced in your Chitta along with it. So that wave represents the idea of the cow, the form or the meaning as we call it. The apparent cow that you know is really the wave in the mind stuff that comes as a reaction to the internal and external sound vibrations. With the sound, the wave dies away; it can never exist without a word. You may ask how it is, when we only think of the cow, and do not hear a sound. You make that sound yourself. You are saying "cow" faintly in your mind, and with that comes a wave. There cannot be any wave without this impulse of sound; and when it is not from outside, it is from inside, and when the sound dies, the wave dies. What remains? The result of the reaction, and that is knowledge. These three are so closely combined in our mind that we cannot separate them. When the sound comes, the senses vibrate, and the wave rises in reaction; they follow so closely upon one another that there is no discerning one from the other. When this meditation has been practised for a long time, memory, the receptacle of all impressions, becomes purified, and we are able clearly to distinguish them from one another. This is called Nirvitarka, concentration without question.

44. *By this process, (the concentrations) with discrimination and without discrimination, whose objects are finer, are (also) explained.*

A process similar to the preceding is applied again; only, the objects to be taken up in the former meditations are gross; in this they are fine.

45. *The finer objects end with the Pradhana.*

The gross objects are only the elements and everything manufactured out of them. The fine objects begin with the Tanmatras or fine particles. The organs, the mind,[1] egoism, the mind stuff (the cause of all manifestation), the equilibrium state of Sattva, Rajas, and Tamas materials—called Pradhana (chief), Prakriti (nature), or Avyakta (unmanifest)—are all included within the category of fine objects, the Purusha (the Soul) alone being excepted.

46. *These concentrations are with seed.*

These do not destroy the seeds of past actions, and thus cannot give liberation, but what they bring to the Yogi is stated in the following aphorism.

47. *The concentration "without discrimination" being purified, the Chitta becomes firmly fixed.*

48. *The knowledge in that is called "filled with Truth".*

The next aphorism will explain this.

49. *The knowledge that is gained from testimony and inference is about common objects. That from the Samadhi just mentioned is of a much higher order, being able to penetrate where inference and testimony cannot go.*

The idea is that we have to get our knowledge of ordinary objects by direct perception, and by inference therefrom, and from testimony of people who are competent. By "people who are competent", the Yogis always mean the Rishis, or the seers of the thoughts recorded in the scriptures—the Vedas. According to them, the only proof of the scriptures is that they were the testimony of competent persons, yet they say the scriptures cannot take us to realization. We can read all the Vedas, and yet will not realize anything, but when we practise their teachings, then we attain to that state which realizes what the scriptures say, which penetrates where neither reason nor perception nor inference can go, and where the testimony of others cannot avail. This is what is meant by the aphorism.

Realization is real religion, all the rest is only preparation—hearing lectures, or reading books, or reasoning is merely preparing the ground; it is not religion. Intellectual assent and intellectual dissent are not religion. The central idea of the Yogis is that just as we come in direct contact with objects of the senses, so religion even can be directly perceived in a far more intense sense. The truths of religion, as God and Soul, cannot be perceived by the external senses. I cannot see God with my eyes, nor can I touch Him with my hands, and we also know that neither can we reason beyond the senses. Reason leaves us at a point quite indecisive; we may reason all our lives, as the world has been doing for thousands of years, and the result is that we find we are incompetent to prove or disprove the facts of religion. What we perceive directly we take as the basis, and upon that basis we reason. So it is obvious that reasoning has to run within these bounds of perception. It can never go beyond. The whole scope of realization, therefore, is beyond sense perception. The Yogis say that man can go beyond his direct sense perception, and beyond his reason also. Man has in him the faculty, the power of transcending his intellect even, a power which is in every being, every creature. By the practice of Yoga that power is aroused, and then man transcends the ordinary limits of reason, and directly perceives things which are beyond all reason.

50. *The resulting impression from this Samadhi obstructs all other impressions.*

We have seen in the foregoing aphorism that the only way of attaining to that superconsciousness is by concentration, and we have also seen that what hinder the mind from concentration are the past Sanskaras, impressions. All of you have observed that, when you are trying to concentrate your mind, your thoughts wander. When you are trying to think of God, that is the very time these Sanskaras appear. At other times they are not so active, but when you want them not, they are sure to be there, trying their best to crowd in your mind. Why should that be so? Why should they be much more potent at the time of concentration? It is because you are repressing them, and they react with all their force. At other times they do not react. How countless these old past impressions must be, all lodged somewhere in the Chitta, ready, waiting like tigers, to jump up! These have to be suppressed so that the one idea which we want may arise, to the exclusion of the others. Instead they are all struggling to come up at the same time. These are the various powers of the Sanskaras in hindering concentration of the mind. So this Samadhi which has just been given is the best to be practised, on account of its power of suppressing the Sanskaras. The Sanskara which will be raised by this sort of concentration will be so powerful that it will hinder the action of the others, and hold them in check.

51. *By the restraint of even this (impression, which obstructs all other impressions), all being restrained, comes the "seedless" Samadhi.*

You remember that our goal is to perceive the Soul itself. We cannot perceive the Soul, because it has got mingled up with nature, with the mind, with the body. The ignorant man thinks his body is the Soul. The learned man thinks his mind is the Soul. But both of them are mistaken. What makes the Soul get mingled up with all this? Different waves in the Chitta rise and cover the Soul; we only see a little reflection of the Soul through these waves; so, if the wave is one of anger, we see the Soul as angry; "I am angry", one says. If it is one of love, we see ourselves reflected in that wave, and say we are loving. If that wave is one of weakness, and the Soul is reflected in it, we think we are weak. These various ideas come from these impressions, these Sanskaras covering the Soul. The real nature of the Soul is not perceived as long as there is one single wave in the lake of the Chitta; this real nature will never be perceived until all the waves have subsided. So, first, Patanjali teaches us the meaning of these waves; secondly, the best way to repress them; and thirdly, how to make one wave so strong as to suppress all other waves, fire eating fire as it were. When only one remains, it will be easy to suppress that also, and when that is gone, this Samadhi or concentration is called seedless. It leaves nothing, and the Soul is manifested just as it is, in its own glory. Then alone we know that the Soul is not a compound; it is the only eternal simple Soul in the universe, and as such, it cannot be born, it cannot die; it is immortal, indestructible, the ever-living essence of intelligence.

CHAPTER II

# CONCENTRATION: ITS PRACTICE

1. *Mortification, study, and surrendering fruits of work to God are called Kriya Yoga.*

Those Samadhis with which we ended our last chapter are very difficult to attain: so we must take them up slowly. The first step, the preliminary step, is called Kriya Yoga. Literally this means work, working towards Yoga. The organs are the horses, the mind is the rein, the intellect is the charioteer, the soul is the rider, and the body is the chariot. The master of the household, the King, the Self of man, is sitting in this chariot. If the horses are very strong and do not obey the rein, if the charioteer, the intellect, does not know how to control the horses, then the chariot will come to grief. But if the organs, the horses, are well controlled, and if the rein, the mind, is well held in the hands of the charioteer, the intellect, the chariot reaches the goal. What is meant, therefore, by this mortification? Holding the rein firmly while guiding the body and the organs; not letting them do anything they like, but keeping them both under proper control. *Study*. What is meant by study in this case? No study of novels or story books, but study of those works which teach the liberation of the soul. Then again this study does not mean controversial studies at all. The Yogi is supposed to have finished his period of controversy. He has had enough of that, and has become satisfied. He only studies to intensify his convictions. Vada and Siddhanta—these are the two sorts of scriptural knowledge—Vada (the argumentative) and Siddhanta (the decisive). When a man is entirely ignorant he takes up the first of these, the argumentative fighting, and reasoning pro and con; and when he has finished that he takes up the Siddhanta, the decisive, arriving at a conclusion. Simply arriving at this conclusion will not do. It must be intensified. Books are infinite in number, and time is short; therefore the secret of knowledge is to take what is essential. Take that and try to live up to it. There is an old Indian legend that if you place a cup of milk and water before a Raja Hamsa (swan), he will take all the milk and leave the water. In that way we should take what is of value in knowledge, and leave the dross. Intellectual gymnastics are necessary at first. We must not go blindly into anything. The Yogi has passed the argumentative stage, and has come to a conclusion, which is, like the rock, immovable. The only thing he now seeks to do is to intensify that conclusion. Do not argue, he says; if one forces arguments upon you, be silent. Do not answer any argument, but go away calmly, because arguments only disturb the mind. The only thing necessary is to train the intellect, what is the use of disturbing it for nothing? The intellect is but a weak instrument, and can give us only knowledge limited by the senses. The Yogi wants to go beyond the senses; therefore, intellect is of no use to him. He is certain of this and, therefore, is silent, and does not argue. Every argument throws his mind out of balance, creates a disturbance in the Chitta, and a disturbance is a drawback. Argumentations and searchings of the reason are only by the way. There are much higher things beyond them. The whole of life is not for schoolboy fights and debating societies. "Surrendering the fruits of work to God" is to take to ourselves neither credit nor blame, but to give both up to the Lord and be at peace.

2. *(It is for) the practice of Samadhi and minimizing the pain-bearing obstructions.*

Most of us make our minds like spoilt children, allowing them to do whatever they want. Therefore it is necessary that Kriya Yoga should be constantly practised, in order to gain control of the mind, and bring it into subjection. The obstructions to Yoga arise from lack of control, and cause us pain. They can only be removed by denying the mind, and holding it in check, through the means of Kriya Yoga.

3. *The pain-bearing obstructions are—ignorance, egoism, attachment, aversion, and clinging to life.*

These are the five pains, the fivefold tie that binds us down, of which ignorance is the cause and the other four its effects. It is the only cause of all our misery. What else can make us miserable? The nature of the Soul is eternal bliss. What can make it sorrowful except ignorance, hallucination, delusion? All pain of the Soul is simply delusion.

4. *Ignorance is the productive field of all these that follow, whether they are dormant, attenuated, overpowered, or expanded.*

Ignorance is the cause of egoism, attachment, aversion, and clinging to life. These impressions exist in different states. They are sometimes dormant. You often hear the expression "innocent as a baby", yet in the baby may be the state of a demon or of a god, which will come out by degrees. In the Yogi, these impressions, the Sanskaras left by past actions, are attenuated, that is, exist in a very fine state, and he can control them, and not allow them to become manifest. "Overpowered" means that sometimes one set of impressions is held down for a while by those that are stronger, but they come out when that repressing cause is removed. The last state is the "expanded", when the Sanskaras, having helpful surroundings, attain to a great activity, either as good or evil.

5. *Ignorance is taking the non-eternal, the impure, the painful, and the non-Self for the eternal, the pure, the happy, and the Atman or Self (respectively).*

All the different sorts of impressions have one source, ignorance. We have first to learn what ignorance is. All of us think, "I am the body and not the Self, the pure, the effulgent, the ever blissful", and that is ignorance. We think of man, and see man as body. This is the great delusion.

6. *Egoism is the identification of the seer with the instrument of seeing.*

The seer is really the Self, the pure one, the ever holy, the infinite, the immortal. This is the Self of man. And what are the instruments? The Chitta, or mind stuff, the Buddhi, determinative faculty, the Manas, or mind, and the Indriyas, or sense organs. These are the instruments for him to see the external world, and the identification of the Self with the instruments is what is called the ignorance of egoism. We say, "I am the mind", "I am thought", "I am angry", or "I am happy". How can we be angry and how can we hate? We should identify ourselves with the Self that cannot change. If it is unchangeable, how can it be one moment happy, and one moment unhappy? It is formless, infinite, omnipresent. What can change it? It is beyond all law. What can affect it? Nothing in the universe can produce an effect on it. Yet through ignorance, we identify ourselves with the mind stuff, and think we feel pleasure or pain.

7. *Attachment is that which dwells on pleasure.*

We find pleasure in certain things, and the mind like a current flows towards them; and this following the pleasure centre, as it were, is what is called attachment. We are never attached where we do not find pleasure. We find pleasure in very queer things sometimes, but the principle remains: wherever we find pleasure, there we are attached.

8. *Aversion is that which dwells on pain.*

That which gives us pain we immediately seek to get away from.

9. *Flowing through its own nature, and established even in the learned, is the clinging to life.*

This clinging to life you see manifested in every animal. Upon it many attempts have been made to build the theory of a future life, because men are so fond of life that they desire a future life also. Of course it goes without saying that this argument is without much value, but the most curious part of it is, that, in Western countries, the idea that this clinging to life indicates a possibility of future life applies only to men, but does not include animals. In India this clinging to life has been one of the arguments to prove past experience and existence. For instance, if it be true that all our knowledge has come from experience, then it is sure that that which we never experienced we cannot imagine or understand. As soon as chickens are hatched they begin to pick up food. Many times it has been seen, where ducks have been hatched by hens, that, as soon as they came out of the eggs they flew to water, and the mother thought they would be drowned. If experience be the only source of knowledge, where did these chickens learn to pick up food, or the ducklings that the water was their natural element? If you say it is instinct, it means nothing—it is simply giving a word, but is no explanation. What is this instinct? We have many instincts in ourselves. For instance, most of you ladies play the piano, and remember, when you first learnt, how carefully you had to put your fingers on the black and the white keys, one after the other; but now, after long years of practice, you can talk with your friends while your fingers play mechanically. It has become instinct. So with every work we do; by practice it becomes instinct, it becomes automatic; but so far as we know, all the cases which we now regard as automatic are degenerated reason. In the language of the Yogi, instinct is involved reason. Discrimination becomes involved, and gets to be automatic Sanskaras. Therefore, it is perfectly logical to think that all we call instinct in this world is simply involved reason. As reason cannot come without experience, all instinct is, therefore, the result of past experience. Chickens fear the hawk and ducklings love the water; these are both the results of past experience. Then the question is whether that experience belongs to a particular soul, or to the body simply, whether this experience which comes to the duck is the duck's forefathers' experience, or the duck's own experience. Modern scientific men hold that it belongs to the body, but the Yogis hold that it is the experience of the mind, transmitted through the body. This is called the theory of reincarnation.

We have seen that all our knowledge whether we call it perception, or reason or instinct, must come through that one channel called experience, and all that we now call instinct is the result of past experience, degenerated into instinct and that instinct regenerates into reason again. So on throughout the universe, and upon this has been built one of the chief arguments for reincarnation in India. The recurring experiences of various fears, in course of time, produce this clinging to life. That is why the child is instinctively afraid, because the past experience of pain is there in it. Even in the most learned men, who know that this body will go, and who say "never mind, we have had hundreds of bodies, the soul cannot die"—even in them, with all their intellectual convictions, we still find this clinging on to life. Why is this clinging to life? We have seen that it has become instinctive. In the psychological language of the Yogis it has become a Sanskara. The Sanskaras, fine and hidden, are sleeping in the Chitta. All this past experience of death, all that which we call instinct, is experience become subconscious. It lives in the Chitta, and is not inactive, but is working underneath.

The Chitta Vrittis, the mind waves, which are gross, we can appreciate and feel; they can be more easily controlled, but what about the finer instincts? How can they be controlled? When I am angry, my whole mind becomes a huge wave of anger. I feel it, see it, handle it, can easily manipulate it, can fight with it; but I shall not succeed perfectly in the fight until I can get down below to its causes. A man says something very harsh to me, and I begin to feel that I am getting heated, and he goes on till I am perfectly angry and forget myself, identify myself with anger. When he first began to abuse me, I thought, "I am going to be angry". Anger was one thing, and I was another; but when I became angry I was anger. These feelings have to be controlled in the germ, the root, in their fine forms, before even we have become conscious that they are acting on us. With the vast majority of mankind the fine states of these passions are not even known—the states in which they emerge from subconsciousness. When a bubble is rising from the bottom of the lake, we do not see it, nor even when it is nearly come to the surface; it is only when it bursts and makes a ripple that we know it is there. We shall only be successful in grappling with the waves when we can get hold of them in their fine causes, and until you can get hold of them, and subdue them before they become gross, there is no hope of conquering any passion perfectly. To control our passions we have to control them at their very roots; then alone shall we be able to burn out their very seeds. As fried seeds thrown into the ground will never come up, so these passions will never arise.

10. *The fine Sanskaras are to be conquered by resolving them into their causal state.*

Sanskaras are the subtle impressions that manifest themselves into gross forms later on. How are these fine Sanskaras to be controlled?—By resolving the effect into its cause. When the Chitta, which is an effect, is resolved into its cause, Asmita, or egoism, then only the fine impressions die along with it. Meditation cannot destroy these.

11. *By meditation, their (gross) modifications are to be rejected.*

Meditation is one of the great means of controlling the rising of these waves. By meditation you can make the mind subdue these waves, and if you go on practising meditation for days, and months, and years, until it has become a habit, until it will come in spite of yourself, anger and hatred will be controlled and checked.

12. *The "receptacle of works" has its root in these pain-bearing obstructions, and their experience is in this visible life, or in the unseen life.*

By the "receptacle of works" is meant the sum total of Sanskaras. Whatever work we do, the mind is thrown into a wave, and after the work is finished, we think the wave is gone. No. It has only become fine, but it is still there. When we try to remember the work, it comes up again and becomes a wave. So it was there; if not, there would not have been memory. Thus every action, every thought, good or bad, just goes down and becomes fine, and is there stored up. Both happy and unhappy thoughts are called pain-bearing obstructions, because according to the Yogis, they, in the long run, bring pain. All happiness which comes from the senses will, eventually, bring pain. All enjoyment will make us thirst for more, and that brings pain as its result. There is no limit to man's desires; he goes on desiring, and when he comes to a point where desire cannot be fulfilled, the result is pain. Therefore the Yogis regard the sum total of the impressions, good or evil, as pain-bearing obstructions; they obstruct the way to freedom of the Soul.

It is the same with the Sanskaras, the fine roots of all our works; they are the causes which will again bring effects, either in this life, or in the lives to come. In exceptional cases when these Sanskaras are very strong, they bear fruit quickly; exceptional acts of wickedness, or of goodness, bring their fruits even in this life. The Yogis hold that men who are able to acquire a tremendous power of good Sanskaras do not have to die, but, even in this life, can change their bodies into god bodies. There are several such cases mentioned by the Yogis in their books. These men change the very material of their bodies; they rearrange the molecules in such fashion that they have no more sickness, and what we call death does not come to them. Why should not this be? The physiological meaning of food is assimilation of energy from the sun. The energy has reached the plant, the plant is eaten by an animal, and the animal by man. The science of it is that we take so much energy from the sun, and make it part of ourselves. That being the case, why should there be only one way of assimilating energy? The plant's way is not the same as ours; the earth's process of assimilating energy differs from our own. But all assimilate energy in some form or other. The Yogis say that they are able to assimilate energy by the power of the mind alone, that they can draw in as much of it as they desire without recourse to the ordinary methods. As a spider makes its web out of its own substance, stance, and becomes bound in it, and cannot go anywhere except along the lines of that web, so we have projected out of our own substance this network called the nerves, and we cannot work except through the channels of those nerves. The Yogi says we need not be bound by that.

Similarly, we can send electricity to any part of the world, but we have to send it by means of wires. Nature can send a vast mass of electricity without any wires at all. Why cannot we do the same? We can send mental electricity. What we call mind is very much the same as electricity. It is clear that this nerve fluid has some amount of electricity, because it is polarized, and it answers all electrical directions. We can only send our electricity through these nerve channels. Why not send the mental electricity without this aid? The Yogis say it is perfectly possible and practicable, and that when you can do that you will work all over the universe. You will be able to work with anybody anywhere, without the help of the nervous system. When the soul is acting through these channels, we say a man is living, and when these cease to work, a man is said to be dead. But when a man is able to act either with or without these channels, birth and death will have no meaning for him. All the bodies in the universe are made up of Tanmatras, their difference lies in the arrangement of the latter. If you are the arranger, you can arrange a body in one way or another. Who makes up this body but you? Who eats the food? If another ate the food for you, you would not live long. Who makes the blood out of food? You, certainly. Who purifies the blood, and sends it through the veins? You. We are the masters of the body, and we live in it. Only we have lost the knowledge of how to rejuvenate it. We have become automatic, degenerate. We have forgotten the process of arranging its molecules. So, what we do automatically has to be done knowingly. We are the masters and we have to regulate that arrangement; and as soon as we can do that, we shall be able to rejuvenate just as we like, and then we shall have neither birth nor disease nor death.

13. *The root being there, the fruition comes (in the form of) species, life, and experience of pleasure and pain.*

The roots, the causes, the Sanskaras being there, they manifest and form the effects. The cause dying down becomes the effect: the effect getting subtler becomes the cause of the next effect. A tree bears a seed, which becomes the cause of another tree, and so on. All our works now are the effects of past Sanskaras; again, these works becoming Sanskaras will be the causes of future actions, and thus we go on. So this aphorism says that the cause being there, the fruit must come, in the form of species of beings; one will be a man, another an angel, another an animal, another a demon. Then there are different effects of Karma in life. One man lives fifty years, another a hundred, another dies in two years, and never attains maturity; all these differences in life are regulated by past Karma. One man is born, as it were, for pleasure; if he buries himself in a forest, pleasure will follow him there. Another man, wherever he goes, is followed by pain; everything becomes painful for him. It is the result of their own past. According to the philosophy of the Yogis all virtuous actions bring pleasure, and all vicious actions bring pain. Any man who does wicked deeds is sure to reap their fruit in the form of pain.

14. *They bear fruit as pleasure or pain, caused by virtue or vice.*

15. *To the discriminating, all is, as it were, painful on account of everything bringing pain either as consequence, or*

*as anticipation of loss of happiness, or as fresh craving arising from impressions of happiness, and also as counteraction of qualities.*

The Yogis say that the man who has discriminating powers, the man of good sense, sees through all that are called pleasure and pain, and knows that they come to all, and that one follows and melts into the other; he sees that men follow an ignis fatuus all their lives, and never succeed in fulfilling their desires. The great King Yudhishthira once said that the most wonderful thing in life is that every moment we see people dying around us, and yet we think we shall never die. Surrounded by fools on every side, we think we are the only exceptions, the only learned men. Surrounded by all sorts of experiences of fickleness, we think our love is the only lasting love. How can that be? Even love is selfish, and the Yogi says that in the end we shall find that even the love of husbands and wives, and children and friends, slowly decays. Decadence seizes everything in this life. It is only when everything, even love, fails, that, with a flash, man finds out how vain, how dreamlike is this world.

Then he catches a glimpse of Vairagya (renunciation), catches a glimpse of the beyond. It is only by giving up this world that the other comes; never through holding on to this one. Never yet was there a great soul who had not to reject sense pleasures and enjoyments to acquire his greatness. The cause of misery is the clash between the different forces of nature, one dragging one way, and another dragging another, rendering permanent happiness impossible.

16. *The misery which is not yet come is to be avoided.*

Some Karma we have worked out already, some we are working out now in the present, and some are waiting to bear fruit in the future. The first kind is past and gone. The second we will have to work out, and it is only that which is waiting to bear fruit in the future that we can conquer and control, towards which end all our forces should be directed. This is what Patanjali means when he says that Sanskaras are to be controlled by resolving them into their causal state (II. 10).

17. *The cause of that which is to be avoided is the junction of the seer and the seen.*

Who is the seer? The Self of man, the Purusha. What is the seen? The whole of nature beginning with the mind, down to gross matter. All pleasure and pain arise from the junction between this Purusha and the mind. The Purusha, you must remember, according to this philosophy, is pure; when joined to nature, it appears to feel pleasure or pain by reflection.

18. *The experienced is composed of elements and organs, is of the nature of illumination, action, and inertia, and is for the purpose of experience and release (of the experiencer).*

The experienced, that is nature, is composed of elements and organs—the elements, gross and fine, which compose the whole of nature, and the organs of the senses, mind, etc.—and is of the nature of illumination (Sattva), action (Rajas), and inertia (Tamas). What is the purpose of the whole of nature? That the Purusha may gain experience. The Purusha has, as it were, forgotten its mighty, godly nature. There is a story that the king of the gods, Indra, once became a pig, wallowing in mire; he had a she-pig, and a lot of baby pigs, and was very happy. Then some gods saw his plight, and came to him, and told him, "You are the king of the gods, you have all the gods under your command. Why are you here?" But Indra said, "Never mind; I am all right here; I do not care for heaven, while I have this sow and these little pigs." The poor gods were at their wits' end. After a time they decided to slay all the pigs one after another. When all were dead, Indra began to weep and mourn. Then the gods ripped his pig body open and he came out of it, and began to laugh, when he realized what a hideous dream he had had—he, the king of the gods, to have become a pig, and to think that that pig life was the only life! Not only so, but to have wanted the whole universe to come into the pig life! The Purusha, when it identifies itself with nature, forgets that it is pure and infinite. The Purusha does not love, it is love itself. It does not exist, it is existence itself. The Soul does not know, it is knowledge itself. It is a mistake to say the Soul loves, exists, or knows. Love, existence, and knowledge are not the qualities of the Purusha, but its essence. When they get reflected upon something, you may call them the qualities of that something. They are not the qualities but the essence of the Purusha, the great Atman, the Infinite Being, without birth or death, established in its own glory. It appears to have become so degenerate that if you approach to tell it, "You are not a pig", it begins to squeal and bite.

Thus is it with us all in this Maya, this dream world, where it is all misery, weeping and crying, where a few golden balls are rolled, and the world scrambles after them. You were never bound by laws, nature never had a bond for you. That is what the Yogi tells you. Have patience to learn it. And the Yogi shows how, by junction with nature, and identifying itself with the mind and the world, the Purusha thinks itself miserable. Then the Yogi goes on to show you that the way out is through experience. You have to get all this experience, but finish it quickly. We have placed ourselves in this net, and will have to get out. We have got ourselves caught in the trap, and we will have to work out our freedom. So get this experience of husbands, and wives, and friends, and little loves; you will get through them safely if you never forget what you really are. Never forget this is only a momentary state, and that we have to pass through it. Experience is the one great teacher—experience of pleasure and pain—but know it is only experience. It leads, step by step, to that state where all things become small, and the Purusha so great that the whole universe seems as a drop in the ocean and falls off by its own nothingness. We have to go through different experiences, but let us never forget the ideal.

19. *The states of the qualities are the defined, the undefined, the indicated only, and the signless.*

The system of Yoga is built entirely on the philosophy of the Sankhyas, as I told you before, and here again I shall remind you of the cosmology of the Sankhya philosophy. According to the Sankhyas, nature is both the material and the efficient cause of the universe. In nature there are three sorts of materials, the Sattva, the Rajas, and the Tamas. The Tamas material is all that is dark, all that is ignorant and heavy. The Rajas is activity. The Sattva is calmness, light. Nature, before creation, is called by them Avyakta, undefined, or indiscrete; that is, in which there is no distinction of form or name, a state in which these three materials are held in perfect balance. Then the balance is disturbed, the three materials begin to mingle in various fashions, and the result is the universe. In every man, also, these three materials exist. When the Sattva material prevails, knowledge comes; when Rajas, activity; and when Tamas, darkness, lassitude, idleness and ignorance. According to the Sankhya theory, the highest manifestation of nature, consisting of the three materials, is what they call Mahat or intelligence, universal intelligence, of which each human intellect is a part. In the Sankhya psychology there is a sharp distinction between Manas, the mind function, and the function of the Buddhi, intellect. The mind function is simply to collect and carry impressions and present them to the Buddhi, the individual Mahat, which determines upon it. Out of Mahat comes egoism, out of which again come the fine materials. The fine materials combine and become the gross materials outside—the external universe. The claim of the Sankhya philosophy is that beginning with the intellect down to a block of stone, all is the product of one substance, different only as finer to grosser states of existence. The finer is the cause, and the grosser is the effect. According to the Sankhya philosophy, beyond the whole of nature is the Purusha, which is not material at all. Purusha is not at all similar to anything else, either Buddhi, or mind, or the Tanmatras, or the gross materials. It is not akin to any one of these, it is entirely separate, entirely different in its nature, and from this they argue that the Purusha must be immortal, because it is not the result of combination. That which is not the result of combination cannot die. The Purushas or souls are infinite in number.

Now we shall understand the aphorism that the states of the qualities are defined, undefined, indicated only, and signless. By the "defined" are meant the gross elements, which we can sense. By the "undefined" are meant the very fine materials, the Tanmatras, which cannot be sensed by ordinary men. If you practise Yoga, however, says Patanjali, after a while your perceptions will become so fine that you will actually see the Tanmatras. For instance, you have heard how every man has a certain light about him; every living being emits a certain light, and this, he says, can be seen by the Yogi. We do not all see it, but we all throw out these Tanmatras, just as a flower continuously sends out fine particles which enable us to smell it. Every day of our lives we throw out a mass of good or evil, and everywhere we go to the atmosphere is full of these materials. That is how there came to the human mind, unconsciously, the idea of building temples and churches. Why should man build churches in which to worship God? Why not worship Him anywhere? Even if he did not know the reason, man found that the place where people worshipped God became full of good Tanmatras. Every day people go there, and the more they go, the holier they get, and the holier that place becomes. If any man who has not much Sattva in him goes there, the place will influence him and arouse his Sattva quality. Here, therefore, is the significance of all temples and holy places, but you must remember that their holiness depends on holy people congregating there. The difficulty with man is that he forgets the original meaning, and puts the cart before the horse. It was men who made these places holy, and then the effect became the cause and made men holy. If the wicked only were to go there, it would become as bad as any other place. It is not the building, but the people that make a church, and that is what we always forget. That is why sages and holy persons, who have much of this Sattva quality, can send it out and exert a tremendous influence day and night on their surroundings. A man may become so pure that his purity will become tangible. Whosoever comes in contact with him becomes pure.

Next, "the indicated only" means the Buddhi, the intellect. "The indicated only" is the first manifestation of nature; from it all other manifestations proceed. The last is "the signless". There seems to be a great difference between modern science and all religions at this point. Every religion has the idea that the universe comes out of intelligence. The theory of God, taking it in its psychological significance, apart from all ideas of personality, is that intelligence is first in the order of creation, and that out of intelligence comes what we call gross matter. Modern philosophers say that intelligence is the last to come. They say that unintelligent things slowly evolve into animals, and from animals into men. They claim that instead of everything coming out of intelligence, intelligence itself is the last to come. Both the religious and the scientific statements, though seeming directly opposed to each other are true. Take an infinite series, A—B—A—B—A—B—, etc. The question is—which is first, A or B? If you take the series as A—B, you will say that A is first, but if you take it as B—A, you will say that B is first. It depends upon the way we look at it. Intelligence undergoes modification and becomes the gross matter, this again merges into intelligence, and thus the process goes on. The Sankhyas, and other religionists, put intelligence first, and the series becomes intelligence, then matter. The scientific man puts his finger on matter, and says matter, then intelligence. They both indicate the same chain. Indian philosophy, however, goes beyond both intelligence and matter, and finds a Purusha, or Self, which is beyond intelligence, of which intelligence is but the borrowed light.

20. *The seer is intelligence only, and though pure, sees through the colouring of the intellect.*

This is, again, Sankhya philosophy. We have seen from the same philosophy that from the lowest from up to intelligence all is nature; beyond nature are Purushas (souls), which have no qualities. Then how does the soul appear to be happy or unhappy? By reflection. If a red flower is put near a piece of pure crystal, the crystal appears to be red, similarly the appearances of happiness or unhappiness of the soul are but reflections. The soul itself has no colouring. The soul is separate from nature. Nature is one thing, soul another, eternally separate. The Sankhyas say that intelligence is a compound, that it grows and wanes, that it changes, just as the body changes, and that its nature is nearly the same as that of the body. As a fingernail is to the body, so is body to intelligence. The nail is a part of the body, but it can be pared off hundreds of times, and the body will still last. Similarly, the intelligence lasts aeons, while this body can be "pared off", thrown off. Yet intelligence cannot be immortal, because it changes—growing and waning. Anything that changes cannot be immortal. Certainly intelligence is manufactured, and that very fact shows us that there must be something beyond that. It cannot be free, everything connected with matter is in nature, and, therefore, bound for ever. Who is free? The free must certainly be beyond cause and effect. If you say that the idea of freedom is a delusion, I shall say that the idea of bondage is also a delusion. Two facts come into our consciousness, and stand or fall with each other. These are our notions of bondage and freedom. If we want to go through a wall, and our head bumps against that wall, we see we are limited by that wall. At the same time we find a will power, and think we can direct our will everywhere. At every step these contradictory ideas come to us. We have to believe that we are free, yet at every moment we find we are not free. If one idea is a delusion, the other is also a delusion, and if one is true, the other also is true, because both stand upon the same basis—consciousness. The Yogi says, both are true; that we are bound so far as intelligence goes, that we are free so far as the soul is concerned. It is the real nature of man, the soul, the Purusha, which is beyond all law of causation. Its freedom is percolating through layers of matter in various forms, intelligence, mind, etc. It is its light which is shining through all. Intelligence has no light of its own. Each organ has a particular centre in the brain; it is not that all the organs have one centre; each organ is separate. Why do all perceptions harmonize? Where do they get their unity? If it were in the brain, it would be necessary for all the organs, the eyes, the nose, the ears, etc., to have one centre only, while we know for certain that there are different centres for each. But a man can see and hear at the same time, so a unity must be there at the back of intelligence. Intelligence is connected with the brain, but behind intelligence even stands the Purusha, the unit, where all different sensations and perceptions join and become one. The soul itself is the centre where all the different perceptions converge and become unified. That soul is free, and it is its freedom that tells you every moment that you are free. But you mistake, and mingle that freedom every moment with intelligence and mind. You try to attribute that freedom to the intelligence, and immediately find that intelligence is not free; you attribute that freedom to the body, and immediately nature tells you that you are again mistaken. That is why there is this mingled sense of freedom and bondage at the same time. The Yogi analyses both what is free and what is bound, and his ignorance vanishes. He finds that the Purusha is free, is the essence of that knowledge which, coming through the Buddhi, becomes intelligence, and, as such, is bound.

21. *The nature of the experienced is for him.*

Nature has no light of its own. As long as the Purusha is present in it, it appears as light. But the light is borrowed just as the moon's light is reflected. According to the Yogis, all the manifestations of nature are caused by nature itself, but nature has no purpose in view, except to free the Purusha.

22. *Though destroyed for him whose goal has been gained, yet it is not destroyed, being common to others.*

The whole activity of nature is to make the soul know that it is entirely separate from nature. When the soul knows this, nature has no more attractions for it. But the whole of nature vanishes only for that man who has become free. There will always remain an infinite number of others, for whom nature will go on working.

23. *Junction is the cause of the realization of the nature of both the powers, the experienced and its Lord.*

According to this aphorism, both the powers of soul and nature become manifest when they are in conjunction. Then all manifestations are thrown out. Ignorance is the cause of this conjunction. We see every day that the cause of our pain or pleasure is always our joining ourselves with the body. If I were perfectly certain that I am not this body, I should take no notice of heat and cold, or anything of the kind.

This body is a combination. It is only a fiction to say that I have one body, you another, and the sun another. The whole universe is one ocean of matter, and you are the name of a little particle, and I of another, and the sun of another. We know that this matter is continuously changing. What is forming the sun one day, the next day may form the matter of our bodies.

24. *Ignorance is its cause.*

Through ignorance we have joined ourselves with a particular body, and thus opened ourselves to misery. This idea of body is a simple superstition. It is superstition that makes us happy or unhappy. It is superstition caused by ignorance that makes us feel heat and cold, pain and pleasure. It is our business to rise above this superstition, and the Yogi shows us how we can do this. It has been demonstrated that, under certain mental conditions, a man may be burned, yet he will feel no pain. The difficulty is that this sudden upheaval of the mind comes like a whirlwind one minute, and goes away the next. If, however, we gain it through Yoga, we shall permanently attain to the separation of Self from the body.

25. *There being absence of that (ignorance) there is absence of junction, which is the thing to be avoided; that is the independence of the seer.*

According to Yoga philosophy, it is through ignorance that the soul has been joined with nature. The aim is to get rid of nature's control over us. That is the goal of all religions. Each soul is potentially divine. The goal is to manifest this divinity within, by controlling nature, external and internal. Do this either by work, or worship, or psychic control, or philosophy—by one or more or all of these—and be free. This is the whole of religion. Doctrines, or dogmas, or rituals, or books, or temples, or forms, are but secondary details. The Yogi tries to reach this goal through psychic control. Until we can free ourselves from nature, we are slaves; as she dictates so we must go. The Yogi claims that he who controls mind controls matter also. The internal nature is much higher than the external and much more difficult to grapple with, much more difficult to control. Therefore he who has conquered the internal nature controls the whole universe; it becomes his servant. Raja Yoga propounds the methods of gaining this control. Forces higher than we know in physical nature will have to be subdued. This body is just the external crust of the mind. They are not two different things; they are just as the oyster and its shell. They are but two aspects of one thing; the internal substance of the oyster takes up matter from outside, and manufactures the shell. In the same way the internal fine forces which are called mind take up gross matter from outside, and from that manufacture this external shell, the body. If, then, we have control of the internal, it is very easy to have control of the external. Then again, these forces are not different. It is not that some forces are physical, and some mental; the physical forces are but the gross manifestations of the fine forces, just as the physical world is but the gross manifestation of the fine world.

26. *The means of destruction of ignorance is unbroken practice of discrimination.*

This is the real goal of practice—discrimination between the real and the unreal, knowing that the Purusha is not nature, that it is neither matter nor mind, and that because it is not nature, it cannot possibly change. It is only nature which changes, combining and recombining, dissolving continually. When through constant practice we begin to discriminate, ignorance will vanish, and the Purusha will begin to shine in its real nature—omniscient, omnipotent, omnipresent.

27. *His knowledge is of the sevenfold highest ground.*

When this knowledge comes, it will come, as it were, in seven grades, one after the other; and when one of these begins, we know that we are getting knowledge. The first to appear will be that we have known which is to be known. The mind will cease to be dissatisfied. While we are aware of thirsting after knowledge, we begin to seek here and there, wherever we think we can get some truth, and failing to find it we become dissatisfied and seek in a fresh direction. All search is vain, until we begin to perceive that knowledge is within ourselves, that no one can help us, that we must help ourselves. When we begin to practise the power of discrimination, the first sign that we are getting near truth will be that that dissatisfied state will vanish. We shall feel quite sure that we have found the truth, and that it cannot be anything else but the truth. Then we may know that the sun is rising, that the morning is breaking for us, and taking courage, we must persevere until the goal is reached. The second grade will be the absence of all pains. It will be impossible for anything in the universe, external or internal, to give us pain. The third will be the attainment of full knowledge. Omniscience will be ours. The fourth will be the attainment of the end of all duty through discrimination. Next will come what is called freedom of the Chitta. We shall realize that all difficulties and struggles, all vacillations of the mind, have fallen down, just as a stone rolls from the mountain top into the valley and never comes up again. The next will be that the Chitta itself will realize that it melts away into its causes whenever we so desire. Lastly we shall find that we are established in our Self, that we have been alone throughout the universe, neither body nor mind was ever related, much less joined, to us. They were working their own way, and we, through ignorance, joined ourselves to them. But we have been alone, omnipotent, omnipresent, ever blessed; our own Self was so pure and perfect that we required none else. We required none else to make us happy, for we are happiness itself. We shall find that this knowledge does not depend on anything else; throughout the universe there can be nothing that will not become effulgent before our knowledge. This will be the last state, and the Yogi will become peaceful and calm, never to feel any more pain, never to be again deluded, never to be touched by misery. He will know he is ever blessed, ever perfect, almighty.

28. *By the practice of the different parts of Yoga the impurities being destroyed, knowledge becomes effulgent up to discrimination.*

Now comes the practical knowledge. What we have just been speaking about is much higher. It is away above our heads, but it is the ideal. It is first necessary to obtain physical and mental control. Then the realization will become steady in that ideal. The ideal being known, what remains is to practise the method of reaching it.

29. *Yama, Niyama, Asana, Pranayama, Pratyahara, Dharana, Dhyana, and Samadhi are the eight limbs of Yoga.*

30. *Non-killing, truthfulness, non-stealing, continence, and non-receiving are called Yama.*

A man who wants to be a perfect Yogi must give up the sex idea. The soul has no sex; why should it degrade itself with sex ideas? Later on we shall understand better why these ideas must be given up. The mind of the man who receives gifts is acted on by the mind of the giver, so the receiver is likely to become degenerated. Receiving gifts is prone to destroy the independence of the mind, and make us slavish. Therefore, receive no gifts.

31. *These, unbroken by time, place, purpose, and caste rules, are (universal) great vows.*

These practices—non-killing, truthfulness, non-stealing, chastity, and non-receiving—are to be practised by every man, woman, and child; by every soul, irrespective of nation, country, or position.

32. *Internal and external purification, contentment, mortification, study, and worship of God are the Niyamas.*

External purification is keeping the body pure; a dirty man will never be a Yogi. There must be internal purification also. That is obtained by the virtues named in I.33. Of course, internal purity is of greater value than external, but both are necessary, and external purity, without internal, is of no good.

33. *To obstruct thoughts which are inimical to Yoga, contrary thoughts should be brought.*

That is the way to practise the virtues that have been stated. For instance, when a big wave of anger has come into the mind, how are we to control that? Just by raising an opposing wave. Think of love. Sometimes a mother is very angry with her husband, and while in that state, the baby comes in, and she kisses the baby; the old wave dies out and a new wave arises, love for the child. That suppresses the other one. Love is opposite to anger. Similarly, when the idea of stealing comes, non-stealing should be thought of; when the idea of receiving gifts comes, replace it by a contrary thought.

34. *The obstructions to Yoga are killing, falsehood, etc., whether committed, caused, or approved; either through avarice, or anger, or ignorance; whether slight, middling, or great; and they result in infinite ignorance and misery. This is (the method of) thinking the contrary.*

If I tell a lie, or cause another to tell one, or approve of another doing so, it is equally sinful. If it is a very mild lie, still it is a lie. Every vicious thought will rebound, every thought of hatred which you may have thought, in a cave even, is stored up, and will one day come back to you with tremendous power in the form of some misery here. If you project hatred and jealousy, they will rebound on you with compound interest. No power can avert them; when once you have put them in motion, you will have to bear them. Remembering this will prevent you from doing wicked things.

35. *Non-killing being established, in his presence all enmities cease (in others).*

If a man gets the ideal of non-injuring others, before him even animals which are by their nature ferocious will become peaceful. The tiger and the lamb will play together before that Yogi. When you have come to that state, then alone you will understand that you have become firmly established in non-injuring.

36. *By the establishment of truthfulness the Yogi gets the power of attaining for himself and others the fruits of work without the works.*

When this power of truth will be established with you, then even in dream you will never tell an untruth. You will be true in thought, word, and deed. Whatever you say will be truth. You may say to a man, "Be blessed", and that man will be blessed. If a man is diseased, and you say to him, "Be thou cured", he will be cured immediately.

37. *By the establishment of non-stealing all wealth comes to the Yogi.*

The more you fly from nature, the more she follows you; and if you do not care for her at all, she becomes your slave.

38. *By the establishment of continence energy is gained.*

The chaste brain has tremendous energy and gigantic will power. Without chastity there can be no spiritual strength. Continence gives wonderful control over mankind. The spiritual leaders of men have been very continent, and this is what gave them power. Therefore the Yogi must be continent.

39. *When he is fixed in non-receiving, he gets the memory of past life.*

When a man does not receive presents, he does not become beholden to others, but remains independent and free. His mind becomes pure. With every gift, he is likely to receive the evils of the giver. If he does not receive, the mind is purified, and the first power it gets is memory of past life. Then alone the Yogi becomes perfectly fixed in his ideal. He sees that he has been coming and going many times, so he becomes determined that this time he will be free, that he will no more come and go, and be the slave of nature.

40. *Internal and external cleanliness being established, arises disgust for one's own body, and non-intercourse with others.*

When there is real purification of the body, external and internal, there arises neglect of the body, and the idea of keeping it nice vanishes. A face which others call most beautiful will appear to the Yogi as merely animal, if there is no intelligence behind it. What the world calls a very common face he regards as heavenly, if the spirit shines behind it. This thirst after body is the great bane of human life. So the first sign of the establishment of purity is that you do not care to think you are a body. It is only when purity comes that we get rid of the body idea.

41. *There also arises purification of the Sattva, cheerfulness of the mind, concentration, conquest of the organs, and fitness for the realization of the Self.*

By the practice of cleanliness, the Sattva material prevails and the mind becomes concentrated and cheerful. The first sign that you are becoming religious is that you are becoming cheerful. When a man is gloomy, that may be dyspepsia, but it is not religion. A pleasurable feeling is the nature of the Sattva. Everything is pleasurable to the Sattvika man, and when this comes, know that you are progressing in Yoga. All pain is caused by Tamas, so you must get rid of that; moroseness is one of the results of Tamas. The strong, the well knit, the young, the healthy, the daring alone are fit to be Yogis. To the Yogi everything is bliss, every human face that he sees brings cheerfulness to him. That is the sign of a virtuous man. Misery is caused by sin, and by no other cause. What business have you with clouded faces? It is terrible. If you have a clouded face, do not go out that day, shut yourself up in your room. What right have you to carry this disease out into the world? When your mind has become controlled, you have control over the whole body; instead of being a slave to this machine, the machine is your slave. Instead of this machine being able to drag the soul down, it becomes its greatest helpmate.

42. *From contentment comes superlative happiness.*

43. *The result of mortification is bringing powers to the organs and the body, by destroying the impurity.*

The results of mortification are seen immediately, sometimes by heightened power of vision, hearing things at a distance, and so on.

44. *By the repetition of the Mantra comes the realization of the intended deity.*

The higher the beings that you want to get the harder is the practice.

45. *By sacrificing all to Ishvara comes Samadhi.*

By resignation to the Lord, Samadhi becomes perfect.

46. *Posture is that which is firm and pleasant.*

Now comes Asana, posture. Until you can get a firm seat you cannot practise the breathing and other exercises. Firmness of seat means that you do not feel the body at all. In the ordinary way, you will find that as soon as you sit for a few minutes all sorts of disturbances come into the body; but when you have got beyond the idea of a concrete body, you will lose all sense of the body. You will feel neither pleasure nor pain. And when you take your body up again, it will feel so rested. It is the only perfect rest that you can give to the body. When you have succeeded in conquering the body and keeping it firm, your practice will remain firm, but while you are disturbed by the body, your nerves become disturbed, and you cannot concentrate the mind.

47. *By lessening the natural tendency (for restlessness) and meditating on the unlimited, posture becomes firm and pleasant.*

We can make the seat firm by thinking of the Infinite. We cannot think of the Absolute Infinite, but we can think of the infinite sky.

48. *Seat being conquered, the dualities do not obstruct.*

The dualities, good and bad, heat and cold, and all the pairs of opposites, will not then disturb you.

49. *Controlling the motion of the exhalation and the inhalation follows after this.*

When posture has been conquered, then the motion of the Prana is to be broken and controlled. Thus we come to Pranayama, the controlling of the vital forces of the body. Prana is not breath, though it is usually so translated. It is the sum total of the cosmic energy. It is the energy that is in each body, and its most apparent manifestation is the motion of the lungs. This motion is caused by Prana drawing in the breath, and it is what we seek to control in Pranayama. We begin by controlling the breath, as the easiest way of getting control of the Prana.

50. *Its modifications are either external or internal, or motionless, regulated by place, time, and number, either long or short.*

The three sorts of motion of Pranayama are, one by which we draw the breath in, another by which we throw it out, and the third action is when the breath is held in the lungs, or stopped from entering the lungs. These, again, are varied by place and time. By place is meant that the Prana is held to some particular part of the body. By time is meant how long the Prana should be confined to a certain place, and so we are told how many seconds to keep one motion, and how many seconds to keep another. The result of this Pranayama is Udghata, awakening the Kundalini.

51. *The fourth is restraining the Prana by reflecting on external or internal object.*

This is the fourth sort of Pranayama, in which the Kumbhaka is brought about by long practice attended with reflection, which is absent in the other three.

52. *From that, the covering to the light of the Chitta is attenuated.*

The Chitta has, by its own nature, all knowledge. It is made of Sattva particles, but is covered by Rajas and Tamas particles, and by Pranayama this covering is removed.

53. *The mind becomes fit for Dharana.*

After this covering has been removed, we are able to concentrate the mind.

54. *The drawing in of the organs is by their giving up their own objects and taking the form of the mind stuff, as it were.*

The organs are separate states of the mind stuff. I see a book: the form is not in the book, it is in the mind. Something is outside which calls that form up. The real form is in the Chitta. The organs identify themselves with, and take the forms of, whatever comes to them. If you can restrain the mind stuff from taking these forms, the mind will remain calm. This is called Pratyahara.

55. *Thence arises supreme control of the organs.*

When the Yogi has succeeded in preventing the organs from taking the forms of external objects, and in making them remain one with the mind stuff, then comes perfect control of the organs. When the organs are perfectly under control, every muscle and nerve will be under control, because the organs are the centres of all the sensations, and of all actions. These organs are divided into organs of work and organs of sensation. When the organs are controlled, the Yogi can control all feeling and doing; the whole of the body comes under his control. Then alone one begins to feel joy in being born; then one can truthfully say, "Blessed am I that I was born." When that control of the organs is obtained, we feel how wonderful this body really is.

# CHAPTER III

# POWERS

We have now come to the chapter in which the Yoga powers are described.

1. *Dharana is holding the mind on to some particular object.*

Dharana (concentration) is when the mind holds on to some object, either in the body, or outside the body, and keeps itself in that state.

2. *An unbroken flow of knowledge in that object is Dhyana.*

The mind tries to think of one object, to hold itself to one particular spot, as the top of the head, the heart, etc., and if the mind succeeds in receiving the sensations only through that part of the body, and through no other part, that would be Dharana, and when the mind succeeds in keeping itself in that state for some time, it is called Dhyana (meditation).

3. *When that, giving up all forms, reflects only the meaning, it is Samadhi.*

That comes when in meditation the form or the external part is given up. Suppose I were meditating on a book, and that I have gradually succeeded in concentrating the mind on it, and perceiving only the internal sensations, the meaning unexpressed in any form—that state of Dhyana is called Samadhi.

4. *(These) three (when practised) in regard to one object is Samyama.*

When a man can direct his mind to any particular object and fix it there, and then keep it there for a long time, separating the object from the internal part, this is Samyama; or Dharana, Dhyana, and

Samadhi, one following the other, and making one. The form of the thing has vanished, and only its meaning remains in the mind.

5. *By the conquest of that comes light of knowledge.*

When one has succeeded in making this Samyama, all powers come under his control. This is the great instrument of the Yogi. The objects of knowledge are infinite, and they are divided into the gross, grosser, grossest and the fine, finer, finest and so on. This Samyama should be first applied to gross things, and when you begin to get knowledge of this gross, slowly, by stages, it should be brought to finer things.

6. *That should be employed in stages.*

This is a note of warning not to attempt to go too fast.

7. *These three are more internal than those that precede.*

Before these we had the Pratyahara, the Pranayama, the Asana, the Yama and Niyama; they are external parts of the three—Dharana, Dhyana and Samadhi. When a man has attained to them, he may attain to omniscience and omnipotence, but that would not be salvation. These three would not make the mind Nirvikalpa, changeless, but would leave the seeds for getting bodies again. Only when the seeds are, as the Yogi says, "fried", do they lose the possibility of producing further plants. These powers cannot fry the seed.

8. *But even they are external to the seedless (Samadhi).*

Compared with that seedless Samadhi, therefore, even these are external. We have not yet reached the real Samadhi, the highest, but a lower stage, in which this universe still exists as we see it, and in which are all these powers.

9. *By the suppression of the disturbed impressions of the mind, and by the rise of impressions of control, the mind, which persists in that moment of control, is said to attain the controlling modifications.*

That is to say, in this first state of Samadhi the modifications of the mind have been controlled, but not perfectly, because if they were, there would be no modifications. If there is a modification which impels the mind to rush out through the senses, and the Yogi tries to control it, that very control itself will be a modification. One wave will be checked by another wave, so it will not be real Samadhi in which all the waves subside, as control itself will be a wave. Yet this lower Samadhi is very much nearer to the higher Samadhi than when the mind comes bubbling out.

10. *Its flow becomes steady by habit.*

The flow of this continuous control of the mind becomes steady when practised day after day, and the mind obtains the faculty of constant concentration.

11. *Taking in all sorts of objects, and concentrating upon one object, these two powers being destroyed and manifested respectively, the Chitta gets the modification called Samadhi.*

The mind takes up various objects, runs into all sorts of things. That is the lower state. There is a higher state of the mind, when it takes up one object and excludes all others, of which Samadhi is the result.

12. *The one-pointedness of the Chitta is when the impression that is past and that which is present are similar.*

How are we to know that the mind has become concentrated? Because the idea of time will vanish. The more time passes unnoticed the more concentrated we are. In common life we see that when we are interested in a book we do not note the time at all; and when we leave the book, we are often surprised to find how many hours have passed. All time will have the tendency to come and stand in the one present. So the definition is given: when the past and present come and stand in one, the mind is said to be concentrated.[1]

13. *By this is explained the threefold transformation of form, time and state, in fine or gross matter and in the organs.*

By the threefold changes in the mind stuff, as to form, time and state, are explained the corresponding changes in gross and subtle matter and in the organs. Suppose there is a lump of gold. It is transformed into a bracelet and again into an earring. These are changes as to form. The same phenomena looked at from the standpoint of time give us change as to time. Again, the bracelet or the earring may be bright or dull, thick or thin, and so on. This is change as to state. Now referring to the aphorisms 9, 11, and 12, the mind stuff is changing into Vrittis—this is change as to form. That is passes through past, present and future moments of time is change as to time. That the impressions vary as to intensity within one particular period, say, present, is change as to state. The concentrations taught in the preceding aphorisms were to give the Yogi a voluntary control over the transformations of his mind stuff, which alone will enable him to make the Samyama named in III. 4.

14. *That which is acted upon by transformations, either past, present, or yet to be manifested is the qualified.*

That is to say, the qualified is the substance which is being acted upon by time and by the Sanskaras, and getting changed and being manifested always.

15. *The succession of changes is the cause of manifold evolution.*

16. *By making Samyama on the three sorts of changes comes the knowledge of past and future.*

We must not lose sight of the first definition of Samyama. When the mind has attained to that state when it identifies itself with the internal impression of the object, leaving the external, and when, by long practice, that is retained by the mind and the mind can get into that state in a moment, that is Samyama. If a man in that state wants to know the past and future, he has to make a Samyama on the changes in the Sanskaras (III. 13). Some are working now at present, some have worked out, and some are waiting to work. So by making a Samyama on these he knows the past and future.

17. *By making Samyama on word, meaning and knowledge, which are ordinarily confused, comes the knowledge of all animal sounds.*

The word represents the external cause, the meaning represents the internal vibration that travels to the brain through the channels of the Indriyas, conveying the external impression to the mind, and knowledge represents the reaction of the mind, with which comes perception. These three, confused, make our sense objects. Suppose I hear a word; there is first the external vibration, next the internal sensation carried to the mind by the organ of hearing, then the mind reacts, and I know the word. The word I know is a mixture of the three—vibration, sensation, and reaction. Ordinarily these three are inseparable; but by practice the Yogi can separate them. When a man has attained to this, if he makes a Samyama on any sound, he understands the meaning which that sound was intended to express, whether it was made by man or by any other animal.

18. *By perceiving the impressions, (comes) the knowledge of past life.*

Each experience that we have, comes in the form of a wave in the Chitta, and this subsides and becomes finer and finer, but is never lost. It remains there in minute form, and if we can bring this wave up again, it becomes memory. So, if the Yogi can make a Samyama on these past impressions in the mind, he will begin to remember all his past lives.

19. *By making Samyama on the signs in another's body, knowledge of his mind comes.*

Each man has particular signs on his body, which differentiate him from others; when the Yogi makes a Samyama on these signs he knows the nature of the mind of that person.

20. *But not its contents, that not being the object of the Samyama.*

He would not know the contents of the mind by making a Samyama on the body. There would be required a twofold Samyama, first on the signs in the body, and then on the mind itself. The Yogi would then know everything that is in that mind.

21. *By making Samyama on the form of the body, the perceptibility of the form being obstructed and the power of manifestation in the eye being separated, the Yogi's body becomes unseen.*

A Yogi standing in the midst of this room can apparently vanish. He does not really vanish, but he will not be seen by anyone. The form and the body are, as it were, separated. You must remember that this can only be done when the Yogi has attained to that power of concentration when form and the thing formed have been separated. Then he makes a Samyama on that, and the power to perceive forms is obstructed, because the power of perceiving forms comes from the junction of form and the thing formed.

22. *By this the disappearance or concealment of words which are being spoken and such other things are also explained.*

23. *Karma is of two kinds—soon to be fructified and late to be fructified. By making Samyama on these, or by the signs called Arishta, portents, the Yogis know the exact time of separation from their bodies.*

When a Yogi makes a Samyama on his own Karma, upon those impressions in his mind which are now working, and those which are just waiting to work, he knows exactly by those that are waiting when his body will fall. He knows when he will die, at what hour, even at what minute. The Hindus think very much of that knowledge or consciousness of the nearness of death, because it is taught in the Gita that the thoughts at the moment of departure are great powers in determining the next life.

24. *By making Samyama on friendship, mercy, etc. (I. 33), the Yogi excels in the respective qualities.*

25. *By making Samyama on the strength of the elephant and others, their respective strength comes to the Yogi.*

When a Yogi has attained to this Samyama and wants strength, he makes a Samyama on the strength of the elephant and gets it. Infinite energy is at the disposal of everyone if he only knows how to get it. The Yogi has discovered the science of getting it.

26. *By making Samyama on the Effulgent Light (I. 36), comes the knowledge of the fine, the obstructed, and the remote.*

When the Yogi makes Samyama on that Effulgent Light in the heart, he sees things which are very remote, things, for instance, that are happening in a distant place, and which are obstructed by mountain barriers, and also things which are very fine.

27. *By making Samyama on the sun, (comes) the knowledge of the world.*

28. *On the moon, (comes) the knowledge of the cluster of stars.*

29. *On the pole star, (comes) the knowledge of the motions of the stars.*

30. *On the navel circle, (comes) the knowledge of the constitution of the body.*

31. *On the hollow of the throat, (comes) cessation of hunger.*

When a man is very hungry, if he can make Samyama on the hollow of the throat, hunger ceases.

32. *On the nerve called Kurma, (comes) fixity of the body.*

When he is practising, the body is not disturbed.

33. *On the light emanating from the top of the head, sight of the Siddhas.*

The Siddhas are beings who are a little above ghosts. When the Yogi concentrates his mind on the top of his head, he will see these Siddhas. The word Siddha does not refer to those men who have become free—a sense in which it is often used.

34. *Or by the power of Pratibha, all knowledge.*

All these can come without any Samyama to the man who has the power of Pratibha (spontaneous enlightenment from purity). When a man has risen to a high state of Pratibha, he has that great light. All things are apparent to him. Everything comes to him naturally without making Samyama.

35. *In the heart, knowledge of minds.*

36. *Enjoyment comes from the non-discrimination of the soul and Sattva which are totally different because the latter's actions are for another. Samyama on the self-centred one gives knowledge of the Purusha.*

All action of Sattva, a modification of Prakriti characterized by light and happiness, is for the soul. When Sattva is free from egoism and illuminated with the pure intelligence of Purusha, it is called the self-centred one, because in that state it becomes independent of all relations.

37. *From that arises the knowledge belonging to Pratibha and (supernatural) hearing, touching, seeing, tasting and smelling.*

38. *These are obstacles to Samadhi; but they are powers in the worldly state.*

To the Yogi knowledge of the enjoyments of the world comes by the junction of the Purusha and the mind. If he wants to make Samyama on the knowledge that they are two different things, nature and soul, he gets knowledge of the Purusha. From that arises discrimination. When he has got that discrimination, he gets the Pratibha, the light of supreme genius. These powers, however, are obstructions to the attainment of the highest goal, the knowledge of the pure Self, and freedom. These are, as it were, to be met on the way; and if the Yogi rejects them, he attains the highest. If he is tempted to acquire these, his further progress is barred.

39. *When the cause of bondage of the Chitta has become loosened, the Yogi, by his knowledge of its channels of activity (the nerves), enters another's body.*

The Yogi can enter a dead body and make it get up and move, even while he himself is working in another body. Or he can enter a living body and hold that man's mind and organs in check, and for the time being act through the body of that man. That is done by the Yogi coming to this discrimination of Purusha and nature. If he wants to enter another's body, he makes a Samyama on that body and enters it, because, not only is his soul omnipresent, but his mind also, as the Yogi teaches. It is one bit of the universal mind. Now, however, it can only work through the nerve currents in this body, but when the Yogi has loosened himself from these nerve currents, he can work through other things.

40. *By conquering the current called Udana, the Yogi does not sink in water or in swamps, he can walk on thorns etc., and can die at will.*

Udana is the name of the nerve current that governs the lungs and all the upper parts of the body, and when he is master of it, he becomes light in weight. He does not sink in water: he can walk on thorns and sword blades, and stand in fire, and can depart this life whenever he likes.

41. *By the conquest of the current Samana he is surrounded by a blaze of light.*

Whenever he likes, light flashes from his body.

42. *By making Samyama on the relation between the ear and the Akasha comes divine hearing.*

There is the Akasha, the ether, and the instrument, the ear. By making Samyama on them the Yogi gets supernormal hearing; he hears everything. Anything spoken or sounded miles away he can hear.

43. *By making Samyama on the relation between the Akasha and the body and becoming light as cotton wool etc., through meditation on them, the Yogi goes through the skies.*

This Akasha is the material of this body; it is only Akasha in a certain form that has become the body. If the Yogi makes a Samyama on this Akasha material of his body, it acquires the lightness of Akasha, and he can go anywhere through the air. So in the other case also.

44. *By making Samyama on the "real modifications" of the mind, outside of the body, called great disembodiedness, comes disappearance of the covering to light.*

The mind in its foolishness thinks that it is working in this body. Why should I be bound by one system of nerves, and put the ego only in the body, if the mind is omnipresent? There is no reason why I should. The Yogi wants to feel the ego wherever he likes. The mental waves which arise in the absence of egoism in the body are called "real modifications" or "great disembodiedness". When he has succeeded in making Samyama on these modifications, all covering to light goes away, and all darkness and ignorance vanish. Everything appears to him to be full of knowledge.

45. *By making Samyama on the gross and fine forms of the elements, their essential traits, the inherence of the Gunas in them and on their contributing to the experience of the soul, comes mastery of the elements.*

The Yogi makes Samyama on the elements, first on the gross, and then on the finer states. This Samyama is taken up more by a sect of the Buddhists. They take a lump of clay and make Samyama on that, and gradually they begin to see the fine materials of which it is composed, and when they have known all the fine materials in it, they get power over that element. So with all the elements. The Yogi can conquer them all.

46. *From that comes minuteness and the rest of the powers, "glorification of the body", and indestructibleness of the bodily qualities.*

This means that the Yogi has attained the eight powers. He can make himself as minute as a particle, or as huge as a mountain, as heavy as the earth, or as light as the air; he can reach anything he likes, he can rule everything he wants, he can conquer everything he wants, and so on. A lion will sit at his feet like a lamb, and all his desires will be fulfilled at will.

47. *The "glorification of the body" is beauty, complexion, strength, adamantine hardness.*

The body becomes indestructible. Nothing can injure it. Nothing can destroy it until the Yogi wishes.

"Breaking the rod of time he lives in this universe with his body." In the Vedas it is written that for that man there is no more disease, death or pain.

48. *By making Samyama on the objectivity and power of illumination of the organs, on egoism, the inherence of the Gunas in them and on their contributing to the experience of the soul, comes the conquest of the organs.*

In the perception of external objects the organs leave their place in the mind and go towards the object; this is followed by knowledge. Egoism also is present in the act. When the Yogi makes Samyama on these and the other two by gradation, he conquers the organs. Take up anything that you see or feel, a book for instance; first concentrate the mind on it, then on the knowledge that is in the form of a book, and then on the ego that sees the book, and so on. By that practice all the organs will be conquered.

49. *From that comes to the body the power of rapid movement like the mind, power of the organs independently of the body, and conquest of nature.*

Just as by the conquest of the elements comes glorified body, so from the conquest of the organs will come the above-mentioned powers.

50. *By making Samyama on the discrimination between the Sattva and the Purusha come omnipotence and omniscience.*

When nature has been conquered, and the difference between the Purusha and nature realized—that the Purusha is indestructible, pure and perfect—then come omnipotence and omniscience.

51. *By giving up even these powers comes the destruction of the very seed of evil, which leads to Kaivalya.*

He attains aloneness, independence, and becomes free. When one gives up even the ideas of omnipotence and omniscience, there comes entire rejection of enjoyment, of the temptations from celestial beings. When the Yogi has seen all these wonderful powers, and rejected them, he reaches the goal. What are all these powers? Simply manifestations. They are no better than dreams. Even omnipotcncc is a dream. It depends on the mind. So long as there is a mind it can be understood, but the goal is beyond even the mind.

52. *The Yogi should not feel allured or flattered by the overtures of celestial beings for fear of evil again.*

There are other dangers too; gods and other beings come to tempt the Yogi. They do not want anyone to be perfectly free. They are jealous, just as we are, and worse than us sometimes. They are very much afraid of losing their places. Those Yogis who do not reach perfection die and become gods; leaving the direct road, they go into one of the side streets in order to get these powers. Then, again, they have to be born. But he who is strong enough to withstand these temptations and go straight to the goal, becomes free.

53. *By making Samyama on a particle of time and its precession and succession comes discrimination.*

How are we to avoid all these things, these Devas, and heavens, and powers? By discrimination, by knowing good from evil. Therefore a Samyama is given by which the power of discrimination can be strengthened. This is by making a Samyama on a particle of time, and the time preceding and following it.

54. *Those things which cannot be differentiated by species, signs, and place, even they will be discriminated by the above Samyama.*

The misery that we suffer comes from ignorance, from non-discrimination between the real and the unreal. We all take the bad for the good, the dream for the reality. Soul is the only reality, and we have forgotten it. Body is an unreal dream, and wc think we are all bodies. This non-discrimination is the cause of misery. It is caused by ignorance. When discrimination comes, it brings strength, and then alone can we avoid all these various ideas of body, heavens, and gods. This ignorance arises through differentiating by species, sign, and place. For instance, take a cow. The cow is differentiated from the dog by species. Even with the cows alone how do we make the distinction between onc cow and another? By signs. If two objects are exactly similar, they can be distinguished if they are in different places. When objects are so mixed up that even these differentiae will not help us, the power of discrimination acquired by the above-mentioned practice will give us the ability to distinguish them. The highest philosophy of the Yogi is based upon this fact, that the Purusha is pure and perfect, and is the only "simple" that exists in this universe. The body and mind are compounds, and yet we are ever identifying ourselves with them. This is the great mistake that the distinction has been lost. When this power of discrimination has been attained, man sees that everything in this world, mental and physical, is a compound, and, as such, cannot be the Purusha.

55. *The saving knowledge is that knowledge of discrimination which simultaneously covers all objects, in all their variations.*

Saving, because the knowledge takes the Yogi across the ocean of birth and death. The whole of Prakriti in all its states, subtle and gross, is within the grasp of this knowledge. There is no succession in perception by this knowledge; it takes in all things simultaneously, at a glance.

56. *By the similarity of purity between the Buddhi and the Purusha comes Kaivalya.*

When the soul realizes that it depends on nothing in the universe, from gods to the lowest atom, that is called Kaivalya (isolation) and perfection. It is attained when this mixture of purity and impurity called Buddhi (intellect) has been made as pure as the Purusha itself; then the Buddhi reflects only the unqualified essence of purity, which is the Purusha.

CHAPTER IV

# INDEPENDENCE

1. *The Siddhis (powers) are attained by birth, chemical means, power of words, mortification, or concentration.*

Sometimes a man is born with the Siddhis, powers, of course, those he had earned in his previous incarnation. This time he is born, as it were, to enjoy the fruits of them. It is said of Kapila, the great father of the Sankhya philosophy, that he was a born Siddha, which means literally a man who has attained to success.

The Yogis claim that these powers can be gained by chemical means. All of you know that chemistry originally began as alchemy; men went in search of the philosophers' stone and elixirs of life, and so forth. In India there was a sect called the Rasayanas. Their idea was that ideality, knowledge, spirituality, and religion were all very right, but that the body was the only instrument by which to attain to all these. If the body came to an end every now and again, it would take so much more time to attain to the goal. For instance, a man wants to practise Yoga, or wants to become spiritual. Before he has advanced very far he dies. Then he takes another body and begins again, then dies, and so on. In this way much time will be lost in dying and being born again. If the body could be made strong and perfect, so that it would get rid of birth and death, we should have so much more time to become spiritual. So these Rasayanas say, first make the body very strong. They claim that this body can be made immortal. Their idea is that if the mind manufactures the body, and if it be true that each mind is only one outlet to the infinite energy, there should be no limit to each outlet getting any amount of power from outside. Why is it impossible to keep our bodies all the time? We have to manufacture all the bodies that we ever have. As soon as this body dies, we shall have to manufacture another. If we can do that, why cannot we do it just here and now, without getting out of the present body? The theory is perfectly correct. If it is possible that we live after death, and make other bodies, why is it impossible that we should have the power of making bodies here, without entirely dissolving this body, simply changing it continually? They also thought that in mercury and in sulphur was hidden the most wonderful power, and that by certain preparations of these a man could keep the body as long as he liked. Others believed that certain drugs could bring powers, such as flying through the air. Many of the most wonderful medicines of the present day we owe to the Rasayanas, notably the use of metals in medicine. Certain sects of Yogis claim that many of their principal teachers are still living in their old bodies. Patanjali, the great authority on Yoga, does not deny this.

*The power of words.* There are certain sacred words called Mantras, which have power, when repeated under proper conditions, to produce these extraordinary powers. We are living in the midst of such a mass of miracles, day and night, that we do not think anything of them. There is no limit to man's power, the power of words and the power of mind.

*Mortification*. You find that in every religion mortifications and asceticisms have been practised. In these religious conceptions the Hindus always go to the extremes. You will find men with their hands up all their lives, until their hands wither and die. Men keep standing, day and night, until their feet swell, and if they live, the legs become so stiff in this position that they can no more bend them, but have to stand all their lives. I once saw a man who had kept his hands raised in this way, and I asked him how it felt when he did it first. He said it was awful torture. It was such torture that he had to go to a river and put himself in water, and that allayed the pain for a little while. After a month he did not suffer much. Through such practices powers (Siddhis) can be attained.

*Concentration*. Concentration is Samadhi, and that is Yoga proper; that is the principal theme of this science, and it is the highest means. The preceding ones are only secondary, and we cannot attain to the highest through them. Samadhi is the means through which we can gain anything and everything, mental, moral, or spiritual.

2. *The change into another species is by the filling in of nature.*

Patanjali has advanced the proposition that these powers come by birth, sometimes by chemical means, or through mortification. He also admits that this body can be kept for any length of time. Now he goes on to state what is the cause of the change of the body into another species. He says this is done by the filling in of nature, which he explains in the next aphorism.

3. *Good and bad deeds are not the direct causes in the transformations of nature, but they act as breakers of obstacles to the evolutions of nature, as a farmer breaks the obstacles to the course of water, which then runs down by its own nature.*

The water for irrigation of fields is already in the canal, only shut in by gates. The farmer opens these gates, and the water flows in by itself, by the law of gravitation. So all progress and power are already in every man; perfection is man's nature, only it is barred in and prevented from taking its proper course. If anyone can take the bar off, in rushes nature. Then the man attains the powers which are his already. Those we call wicked become saints, as soon as the bar is broken and nature rushes in. It is nature that is driving us towards perfection, and eventually she will bring everyone there. All these practices and struggles to become religious are only negative work, to take off the bars, and open the doors to that perfection which is our birthright, our nature.

Today the evolution theory of the ancient Yogis will be better understood in the light of modern research. And yet the theory of the Yogis is a better explanation. The two causes of evolution advanced by the moderns, viz. sexual selection and survival of the fittest, are inadequate. Suppose human knowledge to have advanced so much as to eliminate competition, both from the function of acquiring physical sustenance and of acquiring a mate. Then, according to the moderns, human progress will stop and the race will die. The result of this theory is to furnish every oppressor with an argument to calm the qualms of conscience. Men are not lacking, who, posing as philosophers, want to kill out all wicked and incompetent persons (they are, of course, the only judges of competency) and thus preserve the human race! But the great ancient evolutionist, Patanjali, declares that the true secret of evolution is the manifestation of the perfection which is already in every being; that this perfection has been barred and the infinite tide behind is struggling to express itself. These struggles and competitions are but the results of our ignorance, because we do not know the proper way to unlock the gate and let the water in. This infinite tide behind must express itself; it is the cause of all manifestation. Competitions for life or sex gratification are only momentary, unnecessary, extraneous effects, caused by ignorance. Even when all competition has ceased, this perfect nature behind will make us go forward until everyone has become perfect. Therefore there is no reason to believe that competition is necessary to progress. In the animal the man was suppressed, but as soon as the door was opened, out rushed man. So in man there is the potential god, kept in by the locks and bars of ignorance. When knowledge breaks these bars, the god becomes manifest.

4. *From egoism alone proceed the created minds.*

The theory of Karma is that we suffer for our good or bad deeds, and the whole scope of philosophy is to reach the glory of man. All the scriptures sing the glory of man, of the soul, and then, in the same breath, they preach Karma. A good deed brings such a result, and a bad deed such another, but if the soul can be acted upon by a good or a bad deed, the soul amounts to nothing. Bad deeds put a bar to the manifestation of the nature of the Purusha; good deeds take the obstacles off, and the glory of the Purusha becomes manifest. The Purusha itself is never changed. Whatever you do never destroys your own glory, your own nature, because the soul cannot be acted upon by anything; only a veil is spread before it, hiding its perfection.

With a view to exhausting their Karma quickly, Yogis create Kaya Vyuha, or groups of bodies, in which to work it out. For all these bodies they create minds from egoism. These are called "created minds", in contradistinction to their original minds.

5. *Though the activities of the different created minds are various, the one original mind is the controller of them all.*

These different minds, which act in these different bodies are called "made minds", and the bodies, "made bodies"; that is, manufactured bodies and minds. Matter and mind are like two inexhaustible storehouses. When you become a Yogi, you learn the secret of their control. It was yours all the time, but you had forgotten it. When you become a Yogi, you recollect it. Then you can do anything with it, manipulate it in every way you like. The material out of which a manufactured mind is created is the very same material which is used for the macrocosm. It is not that mind is one thing and matter another, they are different aspects of the same thing. Asmita, egoism, is the material, the fine state of existence out of which these made minds and made bodies of the Yogi are manufactured. Therefore, when the Yogi has found the secret of these energies of nature, he can manufacture any number of bodies or minds out of the substance known as egoism.

6. *Among the various Chittas, that which is attained by Samadhi is desireless.*

Among all the various minds that we see in various men, only that mind which has attained to Samadhi, perfect concentration, is the highest. A man who has attained certain powers through medicines, or through words, or through mortifications, still has desires, but that man who has attained to Samadhi through concentration is alone free from all desires.

7. *Works are neither black nor white for the Yogis; for others they are threefold—black, white, and mixed.*

When the Yogi has attained perfection, his actions, and the Karma produced by those actions, do not bind him, because he did not desire them. He just works on; he works to do good, and he does good, but does not care for the result, and it will not come to him. But, for ordinary men, who have not attained to that highest state, works are of three kinds—black (evil actions), white (good actions), and mixed.

8. *From these threefold works are manifested in each state only those desires (which are) fitting to that state alone. (The others are held in abeyance for the time being.)*

Suppose I have made the three kinds of Karma, good, bad, and mixed, and suppose I die and become a god in heaven. The desires in a god body are not the same as the desires in a human body; the god body neither eats nor drinks. What becomes of my past unworked

Karmas which produce as their effect the desire to eat and drink? Where would these Karmas go when I become a god? The answer is that desires can only manifest themselves in proper environments. Only those desires will come out for which the environment is fitted; the rest will remain stored up. In this life we have many godly desires, many human desires, many animal desires. If I take a god body, only the good desires will come up, because for them the environments are suitable. And if I take an animal body, only the animal desires will come up, and the good desires will wait. What does this show? That by means of environment we can check these desires. Only that Karma which is suited to and fitted for the environments will come out. This shows that the power of environment is the great check to control even Karma itself.

9. *There is consecutiveness in desires, even though separated by species, space, and time, there being identification of memory and impressions.*

Experiences becoming fine become impressions; impressions revivified become memory. The word memory here includes unconscious coordination of past experiences, reduced to impressions, with present conscious action. In each body, the group of impressions acquired in a similar body only becomes the cause of action in that body. The experiences of a dissimilar body are held in abeyance. Each body acts as if it were a descendant of a series of bodies of that species only, thus, consecutiveness of desires is not to be broken.

10. *Thirst for happiness being eternal, desires are without beginning.*

All experience is preceded by desire for happiness. There was no beginning of experience, as each fresh experience is built upon the tendency generated by past experience; therefore desire is without beginning.

11. *Being held together by cause, effect, support, and objects, in the absence of these is its absence.*

Desires are held together by cause and effect;[1] if a desire has been raised, it does not die without producing its effect. Then, again, the mind stuff is the great storehouse, the support of all past desires reduced to Sanskara form; until they have worked themselves out, they will not die. Moreover, so long as the senses receive the external objects, fresh desires will arise. If it be possible to get rid of the cause, effect, support, and objects of desire, then alone it will vanish.

12. *The past and future exist in their own nature, qualities having different ways.*

The idea is that existence never comes out of non-existence. The past and future, though not existing in a manifested form, yet exist in a fine form.

13. *They are manifested or fine, being of the nature of the Gunas.*

The Gunas are the three substances—Sattva, Rajas, and Tamas—whose gross state is the sensible universe. Past and future arise from the different modes of manifestation of these Gunas.

14. *The unity of things is from the unity in changes.*

Though there are three substances, their changes being coordinated, all objects have their unity.

15. *Since perception and desire vary with regard to the same object, mind and object are of different nature.*

That is, there is an objective world independent of our minds. This is a refutation of Buddhistic Idealism. Since different people look at the same thing differently, it cannot be a mere imagination of any particular individual.[2]

16. *Things are known or unknown to the mind, being dependent on the colouring which they give to the mind.*

17. *The states of the mind are always known, because the lord of the mind, the Purusha, is unchangeable.*

The whole gist of this theory is that the universe is both mental and material. Both of these are in a continuous state of flux. What is this book? It is a combination of molecules in constant change. One lot is going out, and another coming in; it is a whirpool, but what makes the unity? What makes it the same book? The changes are rhythmical; in harmonious order they are sending impressions to my mind, and these pieced together make a continuous picture, although the parts are continuously changing. Mind itself is continuously changing. The mind and body are like two layers in the same substance, moving at different rates of speed. Relatively, one being slower and the other quicker, we can distinguish between the two motions. For instance, a train is in motion, and a carriage is moving alongside it. It is possible to find the motion of both these to a certain extent. But still something else is necessary. Motion can only be perceived when there is something else which is not moving. But when two or three things are relatively moving, we first perceive the motion of the faster one, and then that of the slower ones. How is the mind to perceive? It is also in a flux. Therefore another thing is necessary which moves more slowly, then you must get to something in which the motion is still slower, and so on, and you will find no end. Therefore logic compels you to stop somewhere. You must complete the series by knowing something which never changes. Behind this never-ending chain of motion is the Purusha, the changeless, the colourless, the pure. All these impressions are merely reflected upon it, as a magic lantern throws images upon a screen, without in any way tarnishing it.

18. *The mind is not self-luminous, being an object.*

Tremendous power is manifested everywhere in nature, but it is not self-luminous, not essentially intelligent. The Purusha alone is self-luminous, and gives its light to everything. It is the power of the Purusha that is percolating through all matter and force.

19. *From its being unable to cognize both at the same time.*

If the mind were self-luminous it would be able to cognize itself and its objects at the same time, which it cannot. When it cognizes the object, it cannot reflect on itself. Therefore the Purusha is self-luminous, and the mind is not.

20. *Another cognizing mind being assumed, there will be no end to such assumptions, and confusion of memory will be the result.*

Let us suppose there is another mind which cognizes the ordinary mind, then there will have to be still another to cognize the former, and so there will be no end to it. It will result in confusion of memory, there will be no storehouse of memory.

21. *The essence of knowledge (the Purusha) being unchangeable, when the mind takes its form, it becomes conscious.*

Patanjali says this to make it more clear that knowledge is not a quality of the Purusha. When the mind comes near the Purusha it is reflected, as it were, upon the mind, and the mind, for the time being, becomes knowing and seems as if it were itself the Purusha.

22. *Coloured by the seer and the seen the mind is able to understand everything.*

On one side of the mind the external world, the seen, is being reflected, and on the other, the seer is being reflected. Thus comes the power of all knowledge to the mind.

23. *The mind, though variegated by innumerable desires, acts for another (the Purusha), because it acts in combination.*

The mind is a compound of various things and therefore it cannot work for itself. Everything that is a combination in this world has some object for that combination, some third thing for which this combination is going on. So this combination of the mind is for the Purusha.

24. *For the discriminating, the perception of the mind as Atman ceases.*

Through discrimination the Yogi knows that the Purusha is not mind.

25. *Then, bent on discriminating, the mind attains the previous state of Kaivalya (isolation).*[3]

Thus the practice of Yoga leads to discriminating power, to clearness of vision. The veil drops from the eyes, and we see things as they are. We find that nature is a compound, and is showing the panorama for the Purusha, who is the witness; that nature is not the Lord—all the combinations of nature are simply for the sake of showing these phenomena to the Purusha, the enthroned king within. When discrimination comes by long practice, fear ceases, and the mind attains isolation.

26. *The thoughts that arise as obstructions to that are from impressions.*

All the various ideas that arise, making us believe that we require something external to make us happy, are obstructions to that perfection. The Purusha is happiness and blessedness by its own nature. But that knowledge is covered over by past impressions. These impressions have to work themselves out.

27. *Their destruction is in the same manner as of ignorance, egoism, etc., as said before (II. 10).*

28. *Even when arriving at the right discriminating knowledge of the essences, he who gives up the fruits, unto him comes, as the result of perfect discrimination, the Samadhi called the cloud of virtue.*

When the Yogi has attained to this discrimination, all the powers mentioned in the last chapter come to him, but the true Yogi rejects them all. Unto him comes a peculiar knowledge, a particular light, called the Dharmamegha, the cloud of virtue. All the great prophets of the world whom history has recorded had this. They had found the whole foundation of knowledge within themselves. Truth to them had become real. Peace and calmness, and perfect purity became their own nature, after they had given up the vanities of powers.

29. *From that comes cessation of pain and works.*

When that cloud of virtue has come, then no more is there fear of falling, nothing can drag the Yogi down. No more will there be evils for him. No more pains.

30. *Then knowledge, bereft of covering and impurities, becoming infinite, the knowable becomes small.*

Knowledge itself is there; its covering is gone. One of the Buddhistic scriptures defines what is meant by the Buddha (which is the name of a state) as infinite knowledge, infinite as the sky. Jesus attained to that and became the Christ. All of you will attain to that state. Knowledge becoming infinite, the knowable becomes small. The whole universe, with all its objects of knowledge, becomes as nothing before the Purusha. The ordinary man thinks himself very small, because to him knowable seems to be infinite.

31. *Then are finished the successive transformations of the qualities, they having attained the end.*

Then all these various transformations of the qualities, which change from species to species, cease for ever.

32. *The changes that exist in relation to moments and which are perceived at the other end (at the end of a series) are succession.*

Patanjali here defines the word succession, the changes that exist in relation to moments. While I think, many moments pass, and with each moment there is a change of idea, but I only perceive these changes at the end of a series. This is called succession, but for the mind that has realized omnipresence there is no succession. Everything has become present for it; to it the present alone exists, the past and future are lost. Time stands controlled, all knowledge is there in one second. Everything is known like a flash.

33. *The resolution in the inverse order of the qualities, bereft of any motive of action for the Purusha, is Kaivalya, or it is the establishment of the power of knowledge in its own nature.*

Nature's task is done, this unselfish task which our sweet nurse, nature, had imposed upon herself. She gently took the self-forgetting soul by the hand, as it were, and showed him all the experiences in the universe, all manifestations, bringing him higher and higher through various bodies, till his lost glory came back, and he remembered his own nature. Then the kind mother went back the same way she came, for others who also have lost their way in the trackless desert of life. And thus is she working, without beginning and without end. And thus through pleasure and pain, through good and evil, the infinite river of souls is flowing into the ocean of perfection, of Self-Realization.

Glory unto those who have realized their own nature. May their blessings be on us all!

# APPENDIX

## REFERENCES TO YOGA

*These several extracts give an idea of what other systems of Indian Philosophy have to say upon Yoga.*

### *Shvetashvatara Upanishad*

#### CHAPTER II

6. Where the fire is rubbed, where the air is controlled, where the Soma flows over, there a (perfect) mind is created.

8. Placing the body in a straight posture, with the chest, the throat, and the head held erect. making the organs enter the mind, the sage crosses all the fearful currents by means of the raft of Brahman.

9. The man of well-regulated endeavours controls the Prana; and when it has become quieted, breathes out through the nostrils. The persevering sage holds his mind as a charioteer holds the restive horses.

10. In (lonely) places as mountain caves where the floor is even, free of pebbles, fire, or sand, where there are no disturbing noises from men or waterfalls, in auspicious places helpful to the mind and pleasing to the eyes, Yoga is to be practised (mind is to be joined).

11. Like snowfall, smoke, sun, wind, fire, firefly, lightning, crystal, moon, these forms, coming before, gradually manifest the Brahman in Yoga.

12. When the perceptions of Yoga, arising from earth, water, light, fire, ether, have taken place, then Yoga has begun. Unto him does not come disease, nor old age, nor death, who has got a body made up of the fire of Yoga.

13. The first signs of entering Yoga are lightness, health, non-covetousness, clearness of complexion, a beautiful voice, an agreeable odour in the body, and scantiness of excretions.

14. As gold or silver, first covered with earth, and then cleaned, shines full of light, so the embodied man seeing the truth of the Atman as one, attains the goal and becomes sorrowless.

## YAJNAVALKYA, QUOTED BY SHANKARA

"After practising the postures as desired, according to rules, then, O Gargi, the man who has conquered the posture will practise Pranayama.

"Seated in an easy posture, on a (deer or tiger) skin, placed on Kusha grass, worshipping Ganapati with fruits and sweetmeats, placing the right palm on the left, holding the throat and head in the same line, the lips closed and firm, facing the east or the north, the eyes fixed on the tip of the nose, avoiding too much food or fasting, the Nadis should be purified, without which the practice will be fruitless. Thinking of the (seed word) 'Hum', at the junction of Pingala and Ida (the right and the left nostrils), the Ida should be filled with external air in twelve Matras (seconds); then the Yogi meditates on fire in the same place with the word 'Rung', and while meditating thus, slowly ejects the air through the Pingala (right nostril). Again filling in through the Pingala the air should be slowly ejected through the Ida, in the same way. This should be practised for three or four years, or three or four months, according to the directions of a Guru, in secret (alone in a room), in the early morning, at midday, in the evening, and at midnight (until) the nerves become purified. Lightness of body, clear complexion, good appetite, hearing of the Nada, are the signs of the purification of nerves. Then should be practised Pranayama composed of Rechaka (exhalation), Kumbhaka (retention), and Puraka (inhalation). Joining the Prana with the Apana is Pranayama.

"In sixteen Matras filling the body from the head to the feet, in thirty-two Matras the Prana is to be thrown out, and with sixty-four the Kumbhaka should be made.

"There is another Pranayama in which the Kumbhaka should first be made with sixty-four Matras, then the Prana should be thrown out with sixteen, and the body next filled with sixteen Matras.

"By Pranayama impurities of the body are thrown out; by Dharana the impurities of the mind; by Pratyahara impurities of attachment; and by Samadhi is taken off everything that hides the lordship of the Soul."

## *Sankhya*

### BOOK III

29. By the achievement of meditation, there come to the pure one (the Purusha) all powers of nature.

30. Meditation is the removal of attachment.

31. It is perfected by the suppression of the modifications.

32. By Dharana, posture, and performance of one's duties, it is perfected.

33. Restraint of the Prana is by means of expulsion and retention.

34. Posture is that which is steady and easy.

36. Also by non-attachment and practice, meditation is perfected.

74. By reflection on the principles of nature, and by giving them up as "not it, not it", discrimination is perfected.

## BOOK IV

3. Instruction is to be repeated.

5. As the hawk becomes unhappy if the food is taken away from him and happy if he gives it up himself (so he who gives up everything voluntarily is happy).

6. As the snake is happy in giving up his old skin.

8. That which is not a means of liberation is not to be thought of; it becomes a cause of bondage, as in the case of Bharata.

9. From the association of many things there is obstruction to meditation, through passion, aversion, etc., like the shell bracelets on the virgin's hand.

10. It is the same even in the case of two.

11. The renouncers of hope are happy, like the girl Pingala.

13. Although devotion is to be given to many institutes and teachers, the essence is to be taken from them all, as the bee takes the essence from many flowers.

14. One whose mind has become concentrated like the arrowmaker's does not get his meditation disturbed.

15. Through transgression of the original rules there is non-attainment of the goal, as in other worldly things.

19. By continence, reverence, and devotion to Guru, success comes after a long time (as in the case of Indra).

20. There is no law as to time, as in the case of Vamadeva.

24. Or through association with one who has attained perfection.

27. Not by enjoyments is desire appeased even with sages (who have practised Yoga for long).

## BOOK V

128. The Siddhis attained by Yoga are not to be denied like recovery through medicines etc.

## BOOK VI

24. Any posture which is easy and steady is an Asana; there is no other rule.

## *Vyasa Sutras*

### CHAPTER IV, SECTION I

7. Worship is possible in a sitting posture.

8. Because of meditation.

9. Because the meditating (person) is compared to the immovable earth.

10. Also because the Smritis say so.

11. There is no law of place; wherever the mind is concentrated, there worship should be performed.

# NOTES

### CHAPTER I: CONCENTRATION: ITS SPIRITUAL USES

1. The mind, or common sensorium, the aggregate of all the senses. [*Ed.*]

### CHAPTER III: POWERS

1. The distinction among the three kinds of concentration mentioned in aphorisms 9, 11, and 12 is as follows: in the first, the disturbed impressions are merely held back, but not altogether obliterated by the impressions of control which just come in; in the second, the former are completely suppressed by the latter which stand in bold relief; while in the third, which is the highest, there is no question of suppressing, but only similar impressions succeed each other in a stream. [*Ed.*]

## CHAPTER IV: INDEPENDENCE

1. The causes are the "pain-bearing obstructions" (II. 3) and actions (IV. 7), and the effects are "species, life, and experience of pleasure and pain" (II. 13). [*Ed.*]

2. There is an additional aphorism here in some editions:

> The object cannot be said to be dependent on a single mind. There being no proof of its existence, it would then become non-existent.

If the perception of an object were the only criterion of its existence, then when the mind is absorbed in anything or is in Samadhi, it would not be perceived by anybody and might as well be said to be non-existent. This is an undesirable conclusion. [*Ed.*]

3. There is another reading. The meaning then would be: "Then the mind becomes deep in discrimination and gravitates towards Kaivalya." [*Ed.*]